Fibromyalgia Won't Win

Learning, Loving and Living with Chronic Pain and Fatigue

Melissa Reynolds

Author of Melissa vs Fibromyalgia: My Journey
Fighting Chronic Pain, Chronic Fatigue and Insomnia

ISBN:

This book is set in EB Garamond

Cover design and interior formatting by Luke Parkes

Edited by Carrie Kellenberger

Praise for
Melissa vs Fibromyalgia

"I wish this book had been around when I first got diagnosed."

—Deb, a Fibro Fighter

"This book is a very interesting read. It is packed full of information that is easy to understand and apply. The book reads quickly and doesn't weigh you down with heavy text. Melissa is a brilliant writer and I enjoy her work. I recommend her book if you have fibromyalgia or know someone who does."

—Jessie

"Another fine book by Melissa Reynolds. I like that every chapter is stand alone. You can start anywhere and go anywhere. You can read from back to front if you want."

—Danny van Leeuwen, Opa, RN, MPH, CPHQ
Health Hats (www.health-hats.com)

Praise for
Pregnancy & Fibromyalgia

"Lived experience + self-awareness + systems thinking + good storytelling is golden. Add brevity and it's priceless. Melissa's book is priceless."

—Danny van Leeuwen, Opa, RN, MPH, CPHQ
Health Hats (www.health-hats.com)

"Pregnancy and Fibromyalgia is a short, easy-to-digest run-down of things you can expect during a fibro pregnancy, and how to navigate them."

—Diane Murray
Spoonie Living (blog.spoonieliving.com)

"An invaluable resource for fibro baby mammas."

—Caz
Invisibly Me (www.invisiblyme.com)

Dedication

To my fellow chronic illness thrivers and most particularly Stacey, Latoya, Mimi, and Carolyn. What a pleasure to do this journey alongside you. Thank you.

Contents

Disclaimer

None of the content specified in this book is to be treated as medical advice and not as a replacement for a professional healthcare physician. I am not an expert in Fibromyalgia, Chronic Fatigue Syndrome, or Myofascial Pain Syndrome; I am an expert in *my* experience. I share my experiences and research to help you be your own advocate and to make the experience of this illness more visible.

Introduction

Fibromyalgia Won't Win is a bold title. There are many connotations. Some people have very strong feelings around the language we use when discussing chronic illness. Whether one takes issue with the language of battle or not, I hope they see that we all use the terminology that resonates with us. We must use words, especially when we are sharing our stories online or in print.

Every part of my improvement has been a hard-won fight. Each day that I experience just a little less pain and fatigue, I am grateful. My entire life has changed using everything I document in this book. I went from dragging my poor body through each day, hanging on by a thread, to having to continually pull myself back and stick with pacing to avoid symptoms increasing. After having four children in seven years, I am in the best health I have ever been.

I am not finished with this journey. I will never be completely done with self-improvement. I love learning and trying new things, and this book is the enactment of my mission – to share what I am learning in case it helps you. It is not prescriptive; it shares my journey in the hope that it spurs you on in yours, that it makes yours a little less arduous.

I share the key things I do to manage chronic illness and

what I have learnt on the way. Some of it will be familiar from my book *Melissa vs Fibromyalgia: My Journey Fighting Chronic Pain, Fatigue, and Insomnia*. Initially, I set out to update it, and I realised I had edited so much that it was a brand-new creation. I've also added action points at the end of many chapters to help you take these lessons and use them.

We will look at the chronic illnesses in this book, along with the practical parts of my life plan, as well as how to manage life with chronic symptoms.

My journey is intertwined throughout this book. My personal experience makes me a great person to share this book with you, but it also leaves me unqualified to comment on your situation. Every single person with Fibromyalgia presents differently. What helps one of us will not help another. My work is intended to equip you with ideas as a springboard for your own journey.

Let's state something clearly: When I focus on natural methods of managing chronic illness, particularly things like yoga and meditation, please know that I don't mean they are my only recommendation. Fibromyalgia is a complex illness that requires many treatments. Most often this includes medication. I am not a doctor; I can only share my research and experience, and medication is a small portion of what I discuss. As a yoga and meditation teacher and someone who is passionate about the benefits these things offer, I could talk about these topics all day. When I suggest yoga and meditation, it is *in addition* to what your medical team has suggested. These are complementary and supplementary ideas.

I am not healed or in remission. I experience symptoms every single day. My sleep has improved, but it is not near normal. It is still difficult to face my limitations each day, especially when it results in me feeling like I've failed my children or husband. However, my pain and fatigue levels are on average half of what they were daily. My flares are now at the level of my previous daily pain scores. Loads of symptoms are minimal or greatly improved, such as digestive distress, anxiety, and orthostatic intolerance. Brain fog used to dominate my day; words would float away as I needed them, and I would accidentally swap words. For example, I once said "Alzheimer's" instead of "arthritis" when talking to a prominent physician through work and I didn't realise until later. I regularly had bruises on my arms from misjudging doorways.

My symptoms have improved. Most importantly, I have a sense of peace about managing my illness. I can, and have, improved. My toolkit is full of tools I can enact myself, whenever I need. Hope is a shining beacon in the foreground. I believe we will have better answers soon. Research is encouraging in this area. If I could have told myself back then that this is the level of functioning and symptom levels I'd have in my late thirties, I would have been ecstatic.

I hope this book provides you with a sense of hope and a long to-do list so that you can experience improvement in your own journey with illness and chronic pain.

The Beginning

My memory is a foggy one. There are many spots but a few key anchors in my journey.

At 14, I went to the doctor with forearm pain. I was told it was tendonitis and sent on my way with a wrist splint.

I saw many specialists at 17-years-old who gave me the impression they believed I was making it up due to the location of my pain and the intensity of it changing so frequently

Walking down the hill from university in tears due to the burning in my shoulders is imprinted in my memory.

One afternoon, my wrists and lower arms were so sore, I was trying hard not to cry while my mum brought my painkillers to me at work.

One early morning as I tried to leave my house to go to work, suddenly every step became excruciating. It was like something in my lower back had fallen out of place. With tears streaming down my face, I eased into a chair in our lounge to wait for my family to wake up and my mum to take me to the doctor. The doctor thought it was a slipped disc. The x-ray showed nothing unusual. Nothing further was done.

In my last semester of university, I had a nasty virus. It was like a cold on steroids. The fatigue it brought was severe. One shift at the bagel shop I worked at required two bottles of energy drink. In one early morning tutorial, I contemplated using tiny matchsticks to keep my eyes open. I received antibiotics when I went to see the doctor, but I didn't receive an explanation of what I was suffering from. The cold symptoms cleared after three weeks but the fatigue remained.

As I graduated and began full-time work the pain progressed. My neck and back became centre stage. I tried chiropractic therapy, massage therapy, osteopathy, and physiotherapy with dry needling over the next four years as I tried desperately to live my life. My day-to-day functionality was dropping at an alarming rate.

I watched friends progress in their careers, party and go off on their overseas experiences. The true friends were exposed in how they responded to my inability to continue socialising in the same way. It cost me so much just to keep showing up at work. I had little left for anything else.

Somewhere in this time I was given the word Fibromyalgia and nothing else.

It got to the point where I was so miserable, I didn't know how I didn't pass out every single day. I would get up - if you can call it getting up when you barely sleep - in severe pain. I'd get to work with a coffee for the fatigue, then a painkiller that hurt my tummy, and I'd hide in the boardroom nibbling crackers waiting for the stomach pains to pass. I'd watch the clock tick until 5pm. Then I'd walk slowly but determinedly home to the cold flat I lived in. I ate roast vegetables and meat I batch cooked and had over a few days. I'd lie in bed with a hot heat pack and watch a television series on DVD. I was too fatigued to be able to read, which is one of my most loved hobbies.

I went to work when I had my first flu because I didn't recognize the difference between how I usually felt, plus a cold versus the flu. When you get every bug going around, you do not have enough sick leave to stay home for them all.

During this time, I had this hope that if I could work a little less, I might have space to do other things and feel a little better. My doctor dissuaded me saying I'd be disappointed as I'd still be exhausted and in pain but with less money.

Thankfully she was wrong.

Potential Causes

The story of my childhood and my family is a difficult one to share. It is not only mine. There are no villains in the story unless you count alcohol. Like many families affected by alcoholism and addiction, there are a cast of flawed people who did their best.

There is no doubt that growing up in the circumstances I did contribute to the development of my central nervous system overactivation. The disease of addiction cast its shadow over my entire childhood and development.

As the eldest child in a large dysfunctional family, I took on a role of high responsibility. I helped to raise my younger siblings and support my parents.

The one thing we had going for us was love. Despite everything that ever happened, we knew we were loved. And I knew my parents were proud of everything I accomplished.

Once I read *After the Tears: Helping Adult Children of Alcoholics Heal Their Childhood Trauma* (2010) by Jane Middleton-Moz, I was able to see that we were a cookie cutter family of addiction. Our roles were carried out to the letter. It also helped me to process a lot of my own feelings.

There is a decent amount of research on the connection between childhood stress and the development of chronic illness. Trauma can include physical or sexual abuse, neglect, natural disasters, and family dysfunction, such as divorce, parental unemployment, and substance abuse.

A piece of work called the Adverse Childhood Experiences study[1], also known as the ACE Study, is a prominent piece of research that connects childhood trauma and adult ill health. It outlines the risk factors, potential outcomes, and provides a quiz to determine a person's risk of developing health problems. You can answer 10 questions and it will give you your results. I have a high result.

It is good to remember a couple of things. This is not prophetic, and childhood trauma is very common: "*The study's participants were 17,000 mostly white, middle, and upper-middle class college-educated San Diegans with good jobs and great health care – they all belonged to the Kaiser Permanente health maintenance organization. Prior to the ACE Study, most research about effects of abuse, neglect, etc., involved poor people of color who live in the inner city.*"[2] It is not a distant problem, nor is it relegated to a specific socioeconomic demographic or ethnicity.

The quiz doesn't account for protective factors, such as feeling loved, having other supportive adults, and feeling a sense of belonging in your community.

[1] Felitti et al. (1998). *Relationship of childhood abuse and household dysfunction to many of the leading causes of death in adults.* The Adverse Childhood Experiences (ACE) Study. Retrieved from: https://pubmed.ncbi.nlm.nih.gov/9635069/

[2] ACEs Too High. (n.d.). *What ACEs Do You Have?* Retrieved from: https://acestoohigh.com/got-your-ace-score/ (Accessed: 04.03.2022)

The theory is that childhood trauma leaves the sympathetic nervous system switched on. We become stuck in fight or flight response because, as children, we can't run. I will discuss this more in my chapter on the central nervous system.

This is not to say that Fibromyalgia is always caused by these kinds of traumas. It can also come about after illness, pregnancy, and around menopause. We do not know what causes Fibromyalgia. It does appear that we can say trauma is often involved. We also cannot say that by addressing trauma - say, through therapy of some kind - that fibromyalgia is cured.

The amalgamation of the central nervous system overactivation set in motion by my childhood experiences, plus genetic components, and external stressors, such as bullying (which saw me leave school halfway through my second to last year), and then the sickness that perpetrated the chronic fatigue – all of this created the perfect storm: Fibromyalgia.

Not being given adequate help when I continued to present severe symptoms to medical professionals asking for help across a decade (a trauma in itself) contributed to a physiological cascade effect on all systems.

What Are These Syndromes?

At the outset, it is a good idea to define these illnesses that I discuss.

Chronic pain is defined as pain that has continued for more than six months. It can originate from an injury, illness, or other conditions. The pain can range from mild to severe and parts of the body impacted can range from isolated to widespread. Chronic pain can also cause fatigue, trouble sleeping, and it can impact a person's mental health.

A paper from The American Centre for Disease Control and Prevention states, *"In 2016, an estimated 20.4% of U.S. adults (50.0 million) had chronic pain and 8.0% of U.S. adults (19.6 million) had high-impact chronic pain, with higher prevalence associated with advancing age. Age-adjusted prevalences of both chronic pain and high-impact chronic pain were significantly higher among women, adults who had worked previously but were not currently employed, adults living in or near poverty, and rural residents."*[3]

This figure of around 20% appears to be a worldwide average.

[3] Ahlhamer J, Lucas J, Zelaya, C, et al. *Prevalence of Chronic Pain and High-Impact Chronic Pain Among Adults — United States, 2016.* MMWR Morb Mortal Wkly Rep 2018;67:1001–1006. DOI: http://dx.doi.org/10.15585/mmwr.mm6736a2

Fibromyalgia is a chronic pain-based illness of unknown origin with no cure. It affects approximately 3-6% of the world's population. It occurs more often in women than men. It appears to be blind to race, education level, and socioeconomic demographics. The Mayo Clinic defines it this way: *"Fibromyalgia is a disorder characterized by widespread musculoskeletal pain accompanied by fatigue, sleep, memory and mood issues. Researchers believe that fibromyalgia amplifies painful sensations by affecting the way your brain and spinal cord process painful and non-painful signals."*[4]

The key symptoms are widespread pain, fatigue, insomnia, headaches, and brain fog. There are many others that coexist, such as dizziness, paraesthesia (tingling), irritable bowel syndrome, difficulty managing stimuli (temperature, sound, and light).

However, the trouble is that Fibromyalgia seems to be unique to each person: how it presents and progresses, what symptoms are present and to what degree, and what helps said symptoms.

There is also a debate as to whether trigger points are present in Fibromyalgia or part of a separate issue called Myofascial Pain Syndrome. A lot of the above-mentioned symptoms overlap with a lot of different conditions.

Research has found alterations in neurotransmitter regulation, immune system function, sleep physiology, and

[4] Mayo Clinic Staff. (2021). *Fibromyalgia*. Retrieved from: www.mayoclinic.org/diseases-conditions/fibromyalgia/symptoms-causes/syc-20354780

hormone level control. A lot of research suggests that Fibromyalgia is the result of central nervous system dysfunction – specifically an overactive nervous system that is stressing and exhausting the brain (Dennis W. Dobritt, Fibromyalgia – A Brief Overview). I believe that the central nervous system is heavily involved. It is potentially a main factor, but this does not discount the involvement of other systems of the body.

Diagnosis

There are not many people with Fibromyalgia who have a short diagnosis story. A study of 800 patients found it took an average of 2.3 years and seeing 3.7 doctors prior to receiving a diagnosis[5]. It took me several years as the symptoms came on slowly and I was young; the doctors were disinclined to believe me, especially as my symptoms and their severity changed.

It is a tricky diagnosis. Fibromyalgia is often referred to as a "wastebasket" diagnosis. Doctors do have to rule out other illnesses before they can diagnose it. There is no specific test for Fibromyalgia that is widely used yet. The symptoms are generalised: widespread pain on both sides of the body (subjective) for at least three months, fatigue, difficulty sleeping, and difficulty concentrating.

The tender point count used to be one of the defining

[5] Ernest Choy et al. 2010. A patient survey of the impact of fibromyalgia and the journey to diagnosis. Retrieved from
https://www.ncbi.nlm.nih.gov/pmc/articles/PMC2874550/

features of diagnosis. However, tender points were found to be unreliable; you needed 11 of 18 to be diagnosed, and some days, you could have at least that many; while on other days you may have less. You also must find a doctor who wants to help you and believes in Fibromyalgia. I do hope this is becoming a thing of the past, but it certainly was an issue for me.

The medical profession doesn't seem clear yet on whether it is a central nervous system disorder, immune based, neurological, or all of the above. What has been made clear in the last few decades of research is that it is not psychosomatic. However, it is an illness with physiological effects, despite most of the symptoms being invisible.

Misdiagnosis

One issue with Fibromyalgia - besides the difficulty in obtaining a diagnosis and help - is misdiagnosis. One research paper (Fitzcharles & Boulos, Inaccuracy in the diagnosis of fibromyalgia syndrome) puts it this way:

"There is a disturbing inaccuracy, mostly observed to be over diagnosis, in the diagnosis of FM by referring physicians. This finding may help explain the current high reported rates of FM and caution physicians to consider other diagnostic possibilities when addressing diffuse musculoskeletal pain."[6]

One doctor who writes about Fibromyalgia, David Brady,

[6] Inaccuracy in the diagnosis of fibromyalgia syndrome Fitzcharles & Boulos (2003) https://pubmed.ncbi.nlm.nih.gov/12595620/

posits that as many as two-thirds of patients may be misdiagnosed. Interestingly, one of the things that he finds often misdiagnosed as "classic Fibromyalgia" is Myofascial Pain Syndrome, whereas in my case, there is the presence of both, which adds another layer of complexity to these illnesses. Other issues misattributed to Fibromyalgia include thyroid problems, Lyme disease and nutritional deficiencies, as well as other illnesses.

History

Fibromyalgia is not a new illness. There is mention of it under other names going back centuries. In her article *The History of Fibromyalgia* (2017) (on verywell.com), Adrienne Dellwo writes:

"In 1592, French physician Guillaume de Baillou introduced the term 'rheumatism' to describe musculoskeletal pain that didn't originate from injury. This was a broad term that would have included fibromyalgia as well as arthritis and many other illnesses."

And in the journal article *History of Fibromyalgia* (2004) (available on the PubMed website), the authors, Inanici and Yunus, say this:

"For several centuries, muscle pains have been known as rheumatism and then as muscular rheumatism. The term fibrositis was coined by Gowers in 1904 and was not changed to fibromyalgia until 1976. Smythe laid the foundation of modern FMS in 1972 by describing widespread pain and tender points."

What is so disconcerting is that, despite hundreds of years of doctors documenting people suffering from this illness – and my own suffering right in front of their faces – people refuse to believe it. I have been considered lazy and told I ought to 'push through'. The difficulties of fighting this illness were outright ignored.

I am trying to learn to get by without understanding or support, but with the information in this section, I hope that anyone suffering from this illness knows they are not alone.

There is a long history.

There are many people fighting this with you – an estimated 3-6% worldwide[7] – and there is a boatload of amazing writers who share their journey as I am doing here.

Can Fibromyalgia Go Away?
Is There a Cure?

We have been told it is incurable, but that is only because they don't know what causes it. But some smart people are working on it, and I believe we will see progress soon.

There are a multitude of treatment options on offer for Fibromyalgia. Some of them help a little, some help a lot, some help one person a lot and another person a little, and therein lies the difficulty.

I have been sharing my journey for the past decade because

---

[7] National Fibromyalgia & Chronic Pain Association. (n.d.). Prevalence. NFMCPA. Retrieved from the website https://www.fmcpaware.org/fibromyalgia/prevalence.html

I want to help you cut down the time it takes to find what helps you. I have carefully researched, tried, and written about all of the treatment options I have used myself.

Because we are so different, have other comorbid disorders (illnesses that often coexist), and our context and lifestyle are big parts of it, there is no way to guarantee an outcome. But I believe that we can change our quality of life. Otherwise, I wouldn't have created over 300 posts on my blog sharing my journey and turning these posts into tips that can help you.

We must be willing to try things and believe we can improve our quality of life. That gets hard when we get our hopes dashed and the doctors don't even know how to help us.

There are few certainties in treating Fibromyalgia, but here are some:

Treatment will require multiple options (natural and medicinal)

One option can help me incredibly while not helping you at all and vice versa

Sleep is king. Tackle sleep first. Use medication if you must. This is a widely agreed finding from key doctors who treat Fibromyalgia, including Doctor Liptan and Doctor Teitelbaum. (I will share more about these two doctors in due course.) You can impact your quality of life.

But you will probably also need help.

Chronic Fatigue Syndrome

There doesn't yet seem to be an agreement as to whether

Chronic Fatigue Syndrome (CFS) is on the other side of a spectrum from Fibromyalgia, where pain is the most prominent on the Fibromyalgia side and fatigue is the most prominent on the CFS side, or if CFS is a distinct illness. There are a lot of overlapping symptoms.

The key symptoms of CFS are:

- Extreme fatigue, persisting despite rest, for more than six months
- Post exertional malaise
- Sleep problems
- Pain
- Cognitive impairment
- Orthostatic intolerance

I have experienced many of these. Perhaps the most significant, – besides the fatigue and pain,are cognitive symptoms. Losing words, swapping words and short-term memory loss are all very disruptive to life, and especially work life.

Orthostatic intolerance, which, for me, manifests in the form of being dizzy for a few minutes if I stand up too fast because of my blood pressure dropping,can be mild or more debilitating. When I'm more fatigued or unwell, the dizziness can be so profound that I feel like I'm going to faint.

On his website EndFatigue.com, Dr Jacob Teitelbaum, MD, calls Fibromyalgia a 'sister illness' to CFS, and his treatment protocol is laid out in detail. His book *From Fatigued to Fantastic* (2021) refers to both together: 'CFS/FM'. The page on his website discussing his protocol and the research also refers to Myofascial Pain Syndrome.

Myofascial Pain Syndrome

Myofascial Pain Syndrome (MPS) is a chronic, painful condition that involves specific trigger points. The pain can be local or referred. A good definition of MPS that I have come across explains that it is:

"Hyperirritable spots, usually within a taut band of skeletal muscle or in the muscle's fascia that is painful on compression and can give rise to characteristic referred pain, tenderness, and autonomic phenomena"[8].

Signs and symptoms may include:

- Deep, aching pain in a muscle
- Pain that persists or worsens
- A tender knot in a muscle
- Difficulty sleeping due to pain[9]

MPS can also cause difficulty sleeping, headaches, poor mental health, and fatigue.

There is often confusion between the tender points characteristic of Fibromyalgia and trigger points. The propensity for medical professionals to throw every symptom into the Fibromyalgia basket set me back for a decade. If they had realised prior to 2017 that my neck pain was really caused by trigger

[8] Travell, JG, Simons, DG. Myofascial Pain and Dysfunction. The Trigger Point Manual: Upper Half of Body, 2nd edition. Lippincott, Williams & Wilkins, Baltimore 1988

[9] Mayo Clinic. (n.d.) *Myofascial Pain Syndrome*. Mayo Clinic. Retrieved from the website mayoclinic.org

points, then we could have begun working on them sooner. These tiny hyperirritable spots have caused me over ten years of sleepless nights and 24/7 pain that nothing completely relieved. I kept saying that the trigger points in my neck weren't aligning with how they described fibromyalgia. They said NSAIDs don't help Fibromyalgia, yet they helped my neck. They said there was no physical cause of muscular pain in Fibromyalgia, yet these muscles had physical points that could be treated - however temporarily due to the wind up to the nervous system those treatments caused. I was trying to manage two separate conditions (plus insomnia) all alone and they all impacted one another.

This is a devastatingly common situation. Many people with this condition have been undertreated for years. Trigger points are treatable through managing perpetuating factors and treating the points themselves appropriately. By leaving them untreated (or undertreated), patients develop central sensitivity. (More on this below.)

MPS does not have reliable statistics as to the prevalence. Some numbers put it almost universally that approximately 85% of the population will experience trigger points at some point in their lives. An estimate, using data around musculoskeletal pain in general, puts estimates of myofascial pain as a patient's primary complaint at 30%.[10]

The above quoted literature review discusses general treatments for MPS: aside from eliminating as

[10] Overview of soft tissue rheumatic disorders .Irving Kushner, MDSection Editor:Zacharia Isaac, MDDeputy Editor:Monica Ramirez Curtis, MD, MPH Literature review current through: Mar 2018.. Last updated: May 12, 2017. on UptoDate.com.

many aggravators of the condition as possible (like proper ergonomic posture at computers), treating any other present diseases, the treatment usually includes NSAIDS (usually stated as unhelpful for Fibromyalgia), heat pack, and acupuncture applied by a specific methodology.

Some research suggests MPS may develop into Fibromyalgia (see Mayo Clinic). In my experience, Fibromyalgia came first, and then the central sensitivity opened the way for myofascial pain.

Central Sensitization

On the *Institute for Chronic Pain's* website, they define this as: *"a condition of the nervous system that is associated with the development and maintenance of chronic pain. When central sensitization occurs, the nervous system goes through a process called wind-up and gets regulated in a persistent state of high reactivity. This persistent, or regulated, state of reactivity lowers the threshold for what causes pain and subsequently comes to maintain pain even after the initial injury might have healed."*[11]

It's like our brain learns how to be in pain, and it causes more pain. I talk more about the central nervous system in the chapter on Central Sensitivity and Overactive Nervous System.

How I Look at Them

[11] What is Central Sensitization?
https://www.instituteforchronicpain.org/understanding-chronic-pain/
what-is-chronic-pain/central-sensitization

These are just a few of the overlapping pain and fatigue-based syndromes that exist. You may notice that they overlap a great deal.

Most of my coping mechanisms are whole of life (for me as a human being and for symptom management); I look at my body as a whole and try to set good foundations, which, in turn, positively impacts the symptoms I experience.

There are differing treatments for certain symptoms. For example, I need a specific treatment for my neck and upper back (MPS) to function. This is different to the way I manage widespread pain. However, managing pain well manages fatigue well. It also helps me manage sleep better and helps me manage pain in a better way.

I have only just begun to tease the separate strands out in case there is something I can try to help niggling symptoms. Everything outlined in this book will help these conditions and symptoms.

Healing Journey Continued

As I wrote in my previous book, it has taken me many years, thousands of dollars on treatments, reams of paper worth of research, and a lot of hard work to get this far on my wellness journey. I will not stop fighting. I believe I will always need to exert a little more energy than most people to manage my health.

Something I am working on is trying to accept my position as adjacent to 'normal'. I may look and sound 'normal', but my energy levels and pain levels hold me back. Unfortunately, they are invisible, so unless people care to look deeper, they'll never understand.

I have gone from struggling every single day, wondering how I didn't pass out from the pain and fatigue I was feeling, to mostly functioning. And I am profoundly grateful. I didn't want to keep living like that. I will never let myself get back to that. It all started with me taking on the role as head of my medical team, looking at my symptoms like a project and managing them, bringing in expert help where it exists, working with existing resources, and fine tuning as I go.

But it is difficult to accept this box I live in – the carefully constructed walls that enable me to achieve what I do. It is a balance between pain levels and functionality. I must constantly remind myself that I have boundaries and limits for good reason.

It all starts with me claiming the fact that I don't deserve to live in misery. That I can change my life. That it's my responsibility to be as well as I can. I cannot be a good mama or wife if I have not first looked after myself. In a culture of go-go-go living with four high-energy boys, it can be difficult to justify rest, time alone, and all my self-care mechanisms. However, it takes a long time to build back up if I let it all fall.

It took nearly 20 years of coping with the symptoms of this illness, four pregnancies and the first 12 months of baby's life (the most draining time of a person's life) to realise that I can continually push myself. I can dredge through and continue to live with high levels of pain at great cost to my quality of life. But if I fight for it, I can also reduce my pain.

I cannot say if full recovery is possible, but I wholly believe that we have the power to impact our quality of life. My quality of life has improved in such a manner that I am hopeful for more improvement once my children are no longer reliant upon me in the middle of the night or upon my body physically.

2020-2022

The pandemic and adding a fourth child to our family have really taken their toll on me. There has been a lot of change to my health over the past few years. I experienced a heartening level of improvement due to low dose Naltrexone (I have dedicated a chapter to this), and in January 2020, when I weaned my third child, I was looking forward to some stability in my health. At this point, I had a flare up of severe headaches that left me unable to function. This is when we began to realise they weren't just headaches.

In April 2020, I began a new job after being home with my third baby. The day I started also happened to be the first day of the first lockdown in New Zealand in response to the Coronavirus. The person whose job I was covering for their maternity leave was unable to give me a handover as she had her baby before our meeting. I was working 20 hours per week from home on the computer (a perpetuating factor) with no onboarding training, with all three of my children (6, 3.5-year-old and 18-month-old) at home, with no help. My husband was deemed an essential worker and was still working as usual. I was unable to access physiotherapy, which is also a key coping mechanism. It was very difficult physically.

In June, I fell pregnant with our fourth baby, and I had to stop taking my key pain medicines. I experienced the worst morning sickness of all of my pregnancies. The pelvis issues that plagued me through my previous pregnancies returned with a vengeance. This time, I knew how to manage it and was swift to implement all the things I knew that could help. I was lucky enough to be able to get in almost immediately with the specialist physiotherapist at the hospital.

Everett was born at the end of March 2021. It was my easiest delivery. (Easy being a relative term if you know anything about childbirth). We established nursing from about minute 10 and he was a hearty nursling. Unfortunately, he experienced reflux (like my second baby). So, for those first several months, he was uncomfortable most of the time (read: squirmed and cried a lot) and did not sleep. I literally got up with him hourly for most of the first six months. The only way I survived was by co-sleeping.

Despite all of this, my symptoms remained pretty stable. There were periods when the baby wouldn't even nap long enough for a 15-minute meditation and they were difficult. By taking a Yoga Nidra guided meditation rest in the afternoon when the children rested or napped, I got through the days. My neck and back pain levels hovered around 4/10 with flares that brought on the headaches. The headaches ranged from mild to incapacitating. The fatigue was understandably high.

By having and using all of my coping mechanisms, and working proactively with my doctor, I managed to maintain my gains from prior to this period. Though the average pain levels were up a couple of points. I had to relearn how to be more proactive in managing the pain to stop the sympathetic nervous system helping to create more pain.

I learnt something vital in this period - better self-advocacy. I've always been great at advocating for others. I am known for staunchly defending those who need it. But when it comes to myself, I struggle. So, I made sure I worked with my doctor on a pain management plan. He contributed the medicine component and I put in the rest. We produced a physically written pain management plan which I highly recommend you create for yourself. We will talk more about this in my chapter about pain management).

When it was time to discuss my return to work after my maternity leave, I knew in my gut that I wasn't ready and would be unable to cope. We were facing our first Coronavirus outbreak without using lockdowns to manage it. So we didn't know how long our school and kindergarten would remain open in the face of staff and/or child transmission I did not want to send my unvaccinated baby out to childcare. Despite pressure to resume my role as normal, I resisted. And in approaching my boss with an attitude of wanting to come back but feeling like I wasn't ready, we had an open dialogue that resulted in a flexible return. I appreciate how lucky I am to even be able to work part-time in a fulfilling role, let alone receive this level of flexibility. But it is also a testament to the hard-earned experience I have created over my career.

That time I created for myself enabled me to relieve a lot of pressure. For the first time since my fourth baby had been born, my two older children were at school, my three-year-old was attending kindergarten part-time, and so I had days with just the baby. It felt like a holiday. Especially on days the baby napped well, and I could work on my blog, take a decent rest, and get some chores done.

A lot of my symptoms were dormant. The main ones to manage were my neck and back pain and fatigue. As long as I maintained my whole of life protocol, it was manageable. In the rest of this book, I will share more about the key pillars of this protocol.

What I Would Do Upon Diagnosis

When you are first diagnosed with a chronic illness such as Fibromyalgia or Chronic Fatigue Syndrome, your brain has a lot to process. Or perhaps you haven't received a diagnosis yet, but you were nodding your head as you read about the pain and fatigue syndromes above. If you're buried too deep in pain and fatigue, the enormity of the challenge may not hit you immediately. You, like me, may have been diagnosed after a long battle in which you have learnt to push through and assimilate the challenges into your life, potentially making yourself even worse. Or you may have been struck down as if by a lightning bolt of pain and fatigue.

I want to make it as easy as possible for you to improve. Here is what I would do if I started over:

Research

You are your advocate, medical coordinator, cheerleader, and guru. You need to guide your doctor. You need to track your progress. Get a book or open a digital file and write it up. Keep articles that you come across. Because when you're ready, you need to experiment. Your doctor can only take you so far. I highly recommend reading *From Fatigued to Fantastic* (2021) by Dr Jacob Teitelbaum and *The FibroManual: A Complete Treatment Guide to Fibromyalgia for You and Your Doctor* (2016) by Dr Ginevra Liptan. These two authors are doctors who have Fibromyalgia themselves. Their processes are useful and a good place to start. Reading this book counts too!

Prioritise Sleep

Whatever it takes, do it. I have written numerous posts on this on my blog and have a chapter in this book on sleep. When my symptoms flare, it is usually because of lack of sleep or poor-quality sleep. I really hope your doctor recognises the importance of sleep in the body's ability to function. You need to do everything in your power to get enough sleep in order to be well.

Do The Work

There are many types of treatments, medicines, supplements, alternative treatments, physical treatments, and diets. We all have different chemical make ups, different genetics, and different triggers. This means we need to find a lifestyle that helps us live as pain free and as rested as possible.

The complexity of this is huge, especially when you take in the fact that synergies and mixtures of things, may be the solution for you. Your body may need a mixture of medicines, supplements, physical work, and mental work in order to find optimal wellness.

Change Your Lifestyle

Simply put, you can't keep going in the same way. That way didn't work. You need to rebuild your lifestyle and make more time for sleep and rest. Find what works for you, what your passions are (the non-negotiables of your life) and go from there. Try to journal it out or talk it out, or whatever you do to think things through. I spent a long time dreaming of working slightly less hours so that I could rest more and try to recover.

Find Your People

I cannot stress enough the importance of finding online communities that understand what you are going through. Your doctor and loved ones might be the only ones who understand but finding a virtual community will provide you with a tribe of people who understand exactly what you are going through. You need to be exposed to new ideas and you need to be able to ask questions. There are many people struggling along with chronic illnesses sharing their journey. Most people will have brushes with depression/sadness when they're in daily pain and exhaustion, but it always helps to try and keep things positive. Your groups will understand when you need to let off steam and may even have dedicated days that encourage people in the group to share their frustrations.

Start Meditating/Working On Your Central Nervous System

At first meditation was solely for deep rest where none could be obtained any other way. But it's made a huge difference in a great many ways as I discuss in my chapter on meditation.

An emerging theme of treatments popping up is calming the central nervous system and reducing the heightened fight or flight response, often prevalent in Fibromyalgia fighters. As I mentioned in the chapter on potential causes and will discuss further in the chapter dedicated to the central nervous system, this has become a vital part of my understanding of managing fibromyalgia. Although the fight or flight response and stress is important to understand, when you have just been diagnosed I recommend using meditation as a means of rest, taking the side benefits until you are ready to delve into learning about this more.

Summary

This is my core list of things to start with, but really, this entire book is my many years of learning, condensed for you. It's all the things I've done that help me. There are so many more options and ideas out there as long as you're able to keep your eyes and ears open.

Action Points

Start your research. There is good news here: In reading this book, you have already started! Look into getting one of the two books recommended in this chapter.

What Can I Do?
Building Your Toolkit

This is the question and the mindset shift that will change your life. What can I do to make things better today? How can I create a system to make this more achievable? Which health professional can I enlist to help me with finding wellness?

Self-efficacy (knowing you can help yourself) is research proven to improve our outcomes. This study found: *"Higher self-efficacy was associated with less pain and less impairment on the physical activities measure after controlling for demographic and disease severity measures."*[12]

Presumably because if you think you can make a difference, you are more likely to try. It is difficult in the face of high pain and fatigue levels to continually try to make improvements.

[12] Arthritis Care Res. 1995 Mar;8(1):43-50. doi: 10.1002/art.1790080110. Self-efficacy, pain, and physical activity among fibromyalgia subjects

S P Buckelew, S E Murray, J E Hewett, J Johnson, B Huyser
https://pubmed.ncbi.nlm.nih.gov/7794981/#:~:text=Results%3A%20Higher%20self%2Defficacy%20was,pain%20and%20physical%20activities%20impairment.

I completed my 200-hour yoga teacher training during maternity leave with my third baby with fibromyalgia! The beauty of the online revolution is that things like education have become more accessible to people with chronic illness and small children. The 200 hours were completed on my timeline, leaving plenty of time for me to focus on what my body needed and my babies.

There is no cure for fibromyalgia, but there are 1001 things you can do to make your life even 1% better today. Don't believe me? Try something in this book. The first thing I recommend patients try is a Yoga Nidra guided meditation. I have a free meditation you can get on the book page on my website. Do it for 15 minutes every day for the next month. The basis of all my work is the viewpoint of what can be done. What choices can I make to make things a little more manageable? What systems can be put in place to help make things a little easier for myself?.

It also feels nicer to think of all the things you can do as opposed to what you can't do, especially on those days when your symptoms are so extreme you cannot continue with any part of your usual daily life. There are little decisions you can make to improve your experience. A special blanket, a comforting cup of tea, your favourite smells, food treats, and contacting people who will lift you up are all examples of things that can make you feel a little better during hard times. Remember to take your medicine as prescribed and needed.

By creating your symptom management toolkit and your plans you move from a reactive outlook to proactive outlook, and this is always the better front to fight on. This book is designed to help you build your toolkit, from daily management plans to flare plans and more. Approaching all of the options from yoga stretches to medications as tools will help you assemble your coping plans and enact them easily.

When you can anticipate a situation and put plans in place to manage it, you potentially limit the repercussions on your daily quality of life. Once you have your day-to-day systems in place, it becomes second nature to think ahead like this and concoct your coping plans. For example, when I was experiencing a flurry of migraines, I worked with my doctor to make a management plan specific to migraines. This management plan had a positive flow on effects for my general pain levels because a lot of it is connected. So, take notes. use the free templates and all of the resources provided in my book

Action Points

I have created a goodie bag of resources to help you get going with implementing what I offer in this book.

Check out your Book Goodie Bag!

BOOK GOODIE BAG

Pacing and Boundaries

The first active choice I made in my healing journey was to try and use the energy and physical abilities I had more wisely. In moving back in with my parents and younger brothers, I was able to start experimenting with aligning my energy envelope with my responsibilities a little better. By reducing my expenses and having achieved a level of experience that meant a higher pay rate, I could reduce my work hours. I had been working 9am-5pm with a 60-minute commute on a crowded bus each way. By reducing my hours to 8.30am - 2.30pm and driving half an hour each way, I freed up a lot of energy and reduced the time needed on the computer. (This was a big perpetuating factor, which I didn't yet know about). I didn't know it at the time but when I started doing this, I was pacing for pain management. Pacing is a word often thrown about, yet it is difficult to implement, especially if you are trying to live adjacent to normal. Even more so if the people in your life don't understand the consequences if you don't manage your energy well.

The pain-fatigue cycle is a vicious one. You can be exhausted due to high pain levels and then high pain levels lead to exhaustion.

Mounds of literature (and sources) on Fibromyalgia include pacing (see the website *ThePainToolkit.com*) as a core nonmedicinal treatment. A part of what you can do in cognitive behavioural therapy (another prominent Fibromyalgia treatment) is to keep a diary of your activities for the purposes of finding limits and trying to stick to them.

What is the point of this? You're trying to reduce your day-to-day symptoms as much as possible! My biggest aim in life, besides being a good mama and helping as many people as I can with my work, is keeping my   pain and fatigue as low as possible. Using our energy wisely creates more energy. But even if it doesn't, it makes life more tolerable and reduces flare ups.

One of the first things I realised when I cut down on my work hours was that there were multiple benefits to finishing work at 3pm. While I'm unable to keep my brain and body sitting at the computer at this point, they do respond well to a brief rest and then a change in activity. This enabled me to increase my functionality as well as decreasing symptoms.

What has pacing done for me?

- Better sleep - The less overtired I am, the better I sleep. If I've had my rest breaks, relaxed in the evening, and gone to bed at a decent time, I sleep much better than if I don't. (Fun fact: I sleep the worst on days when I haven't rested and go to bed late. Sleep reverse psychology doesn't work here!)
- Reduced pain – By taking my rest breaks and adhering to my framework I experience less pain, especially by limiting computer time
- Less brain fog and feeling overwhelmed
- Better quality of life

A fellow Fibromyalgia fighter, Anne Leppert, shared her tools for using pacing strategies to manage her symptoms in her article *Controlling Symptoms Through Pacing*[13] on the *CFIDS Self Help* website. She focused on things like listening to your body, keeping a log of activities, focusing on sustainability and more. We ought to be emulating her suggestions.

The concept of balancing activity and rest became integral to surviving my first pregnancy. I couldn't physically sustain the crash and burn style I was used to. During the first and third trimester I physically could not maintain my habits of pushing through. My body would send me right back to bed if I didn't listen to the cues. This was the first experience I had with having blocks of time that I was physically unable to continue. I had to lie down and do nothing. At this time listening to *Pride and Prejudice* by Jane Austen as an audiobook was the only thing that saved me as I lay there unable to do anything else. I chose this book because I know it so well that when my attention lapsed or I dozed off, it didn't take any concentration to figure out what was happening.

Meditation has supercharged my biggest rest period in a day – aiming for 20-30 minutes is perfect. I share more about this in my chapter dedicated to meditation. Efficient and proper rest is vital to making pacing pay dividends.

It is difficult to ascertain limits as they change day to day and season to season. But you can pay attention and begin to

---

[13] Anne Leppert. (n.d.). Controlling Symptoms Through Pacing. Retrieved from http://www.cfsselfhelp.org/library/control_through_pacing

keep a note of your activity levels and pain levels. Patterns will emerge.

Boundaries become important once you have recognised your limits and your pacing requirements. Sometimes, you'll need to fight for them.

Here are some tips to help:

- Keep to your desired bedtime, no matter what others may say.
- Take a 10-minute Yoga Nidra or body scan meditation in the car after work and before picking the children up if you are not at home during the day to rest.
- Find a stretch that you always find particularly delicious and do it a few times a day.
- Utilise pacing tools when doing computer work. Always practice good ergonomics!
- Create an exercise plan and slowly work up, allowing for extra tired/painful days.
- Learn that you need to look after yourself. Put that oxygen mask on yourself before you help others with theirs!
- Grab any opportunity to do a meditation/hobby/exercise you love.
- Try to listen to your body's signals and your intuition. But always expect slightly more.

Finding and respecting our energy envelope is crucial to surviving when we have 70, 60, 50 or less percentages of the energy levels that most of the people around us do. For me, this was and continues to be an important part of my wellness plan. I have a free pacing training guide to help you create your own plan. You can find it on my website (*melissavsfibromyalgia*.com).

I like the ME/CFS & Fibromyalgia Rating Scale as accessed at cfselfhelp.org[14]. It aligns symptoms with hours of activity on a scale of 100. It helps to visualise our result as a percentage, especially when we are explaining it to other people. It is interesting as I am about 60% on the scale because the symptom levels here are described as mild to moderate.

There is a big difference in working 6-7 hours with moderate symptom levels and working the same number with mild symptoms! Each step represents a big change for someone's quality of life. For reference, "work" is physical activity. It doesn't matter whether it is paid or unpaid work. For example, when I work in my paid job, I also come home and do several more with the children and house. All kinds of work must be factored in to figure out our ideal energy envelope.

Many of us have little choice about how much we work. I have no choice but to manage these children no matter my symptom levels. In 2021, with a new baby who didn't sleep (reflux issues), plus three other children at home (lockdowns), I had no choice but to do more than even healthy people can do in 24 hours a day. But I paid for it with increased symptoms. I used my work-rest ratios to help me get by. We will discuss rest more in my chapters on meditation and Yoga Nidra. This could be as simple as five minutes rest for every 30 minutes you work.

[14] ME/CFS & Fibromyalgia Rating Scale. (n.d.). Retrieved from http://cfsselfhelp.org/cfs-fibromyalgia-rating-scale

Do whatever helps you manage your symptoms. This is where symptom and activity tracking helps you to assess what your ideal work-rest ratio is. For example, if you can do 30 minutes of cleaning, but it leaves you needing more than an hour of rest and higher symptom levels for the rest of the day, that is not your ideal work-rest ratio. At each juncture of life, we must reassess what our pacing will look like. Each time I have returned to work after maternity leave, I have had to factor in our whole family context when deciding how my work will look. It is a bit like trying to see the future as we don't always know how our symptoms will react and what it's like managing new situations.

It comes back to asking the question, "What can I do?". There are hard decisions to be made when it comes to living with chronic illness. And we must live with the consequences of our decisions. Sometimes we miss out, sometimes we do something and experience worse symptoms. There are workarounds, even for those of us who feel there are limited choices. When I was back at work after my first son, I was exhausted, my symptoms were not well managed because I was just starting my journey, and I had to work and look after a busy toddler. My choice at that time was to sit in my car and do a 10-minute Yoga Nidra meditation before picking my son up from childcare. We can sprinkle in efficient rest stops like this whenever it works. One can always find time to sneak in a gentle breathing practice. I share more about this in my chapter on yoga.

The concept of pacing transcends the macro level work-life ratio, which is also known as how many hours you can be active in a day. It can also be used for the micro, which is the work-rest ratio in a day. The concept of aligning our responsibilities with energy and pain friendly principles is a valuable tool for us.

A note about today's focus on productivity in order to manage all the responsibilities we have: Sleep and rest are not negotiable! They are not negotiable for the average joe, and they are critical for us. If someone advises you to *just* get up earlier or forgo rest so you can get things done, yet you are barely managing the level of rest and sleep you are getting, ignore them. Paradoxically, you will get more done and achieve a better quality if you have rested and slept as well as possible.

Micro Tasking

Micro tasking is my use of pacing in everyday life. As we have established, the concept of pacing is important for someone with chronic illness - especially where chronic pain and fatigue are factors. It simply means using your energy and abilities wisely.

As a person who uses pacing to help me in many areas of my life, and who had a chronic illness before they had children, it's no wonder I apply the concepts now.

I have about 60-70% of a "normal" energy level (and a wonky charging capability). So, I get about six or seven good, productive hours in the day if I am wise about how I allot them.

This is where micro tasking comes in. By cleverly changing up tasks, taking a rest break after lunch (and many other self-care measures) I manage a small business, four children under eight years old and all the rest of the things.

How does one do this (change up tasks, plan their day, achieve goals)?

1. Take your goals.
2. Break them down into key objectives.
3. Break those down into micro tasks.

For example, I am a writer and content creator. But I am a mama first. So, I have created systems for how I create content and get it published, using micro tasks, around my children. I take my pockets of time - particularly 10am each morning - and continue momentum with micro tasks. My master to-do list for my creative work is in Asana. I transfer this to my Paced Planning Journal (available on Amazon), or any planner works. Each day I give myself 30 minutes on the computer to complete one or two tasks from the list. I take pockets of time in the day for my writing. Being nap trapped (stuck under sleeping baby) is for writing or learning (upskilling is important to me). If my husband takes the kids out and I have some time to myself, I know exactly what I need to do. My list of micro tasks is always ready.

Each day I enter the tasks I hope to achieve from the master list (and allot a designation of high or low energy requirements) and add the days paced cleaning tasks (I have a Paced Cleaning Plan too) to the list. I then sketch out my day plan. This day plan always includes my rest break, it's non-negotiable.

What types of things can you break into micro tasks?

- Your health promoting routines and symptom management plans.
- Household chores - you can break them all down into

10–15-minute increments and you can also set a timer and spend 10-15 minutes at one time. I assign one room per day across the week and allow myself 15 minutes to work on that room at a time.

- Business and hobbies (as I shared above).
- Learning - I love to learn so instead of saying, "I'm too busy" - I fit it into my life. This can mean watching a YouTube video or webinar, reading a book, or completing an online course. There are many ways to achieve this. I achieved my 200-hour Meditation Teacher Training program in snippets of time while my fourth baby was small using my tablet for the theoretical components and my daily meditation practice as part of the practical.
- Exercise - my 10 minutes a day series will help you with this (free on my blog), but you can allot one, two, five, 10 or more minutes to this. It can be gentle stretches, walking in water, walking on the street, Tai Chi, weightlifting – whatever you like.

So, what do you need to do?

- Plan well - create a master list of objectives, break it down into smaller To Do lists (monthly or weekly works well)
- Create one time that can be habitual - one 15- or 30-minute time for micro tasking (this gives you your habit and teaches you what you can manage in your time slot, helping improve your ability to break things down into micro tasks).

- Do the tasks! Then take the rests.

Action Points

See my free Pacing training:

Start thinking through your current lifestyle and see what you can add to help you manage and what you can reduce or remove.

Write down what you do each day and track your pain and fatigue levels – look for the patterns over a two-week period.

Use a pedometer or Fitbit or other kind of activity tracker that can be useful for helping you to find your ideal energy envelope.

I provide a free symptom tracker at the above-mentioned link to my blog at *melissavsfibromyalgia.com*. I also have a Symptom Tracking Journal available on Amazon. It's also linked on my blog.

The Foundation Upon Which All Is Built: Sleep

Sleep is the cornerstone, the foundation upon which everything else is built. I've tried all the supplements, all the exercises, stretches, researched relentlessly, and experimented a lot, but full wellbeing is impossible without sleep.

I feel like the sleep disorder part of Fibromyalgia is really overlooked. It certainly has been in my experience with the New Zealand medical system. Sleep is a basic human necessity, yet we live in chronic sleep deprivation.

Insomnia can be difficulty getting to sleep, trouble staying asleep, waking too early and/or being unable to go back to sleep. Sleep quality is an issue with fibromyalgia. Being able to achieve the deeper stages of sleep is difficult.

Sleep Research

Dr Ginevra Liptan, MD, writes about this in her book *The Fibro Manual* (2016):

"Sleep studies show that Fibromyalgia subjects show abnormal 'awake-type' brain waves all night long, with reduced and interrupted deep sleep and frequent 'mini-awakenings'

(Brandi 1994; Kooh 2003). This deep-sleep deprivation leads to pain, fatigue, and poor brain function (Lerma 2011; Moldofsky 2008; Harding 1998). Treatment focused on increasing deep sleep is the key to improving all these symptoms."

In plain terms, people with Fibromyalgia don't tend to reach stage four of the sleep cycle (the deep, restorative stage), and therefore, they suffer from chronic, deep sleep deprivation, which causes all sorts of issues with the body: pain, fatigue, fog, anxiety, etc.

In his article, *8 Tips for Better, More Effective Sleep* (n.d.) (available on the *Paleohacks* website), Casey Thaler explains that sleep deprivation is "very similar to speeding up the process of dying of old age."[15] No wonder we feel like Fibromyalgia is progressive. Until we take the sleep problem seriously, we are exacerbating the aging process.

The research on sleep is fascinating, and I learnt a lot reading *Night School: Wake up to the Power of Sleep* by Richard Wiseman (2013).

What is interesting is that I appear to follow the usual circadian rhythm. My body will start waking up at 7am, peak at 11am, decline to the lowest point by 3, climb and peak again around 7 with my body seeking sleep from 9pm onwards. So, I assume I just have a slightly weaker ability to wake and sleep than others, while still following the natural pattern.

Wiseman references a lot of research. For example, in 2006, it was *"estimated that around sixty million Americans suffer*

[15] Casey Thaler. (n.d.) *8 Tips for Better, More Effective* Sleep. Retrieved from https://blog.paleohacks.com/how-to-sleep-better/

from a chronic sleep disorder" (p. 57) and approximately a third of Americans now get less than seven hours of sleep per night. In a British study, more than 30% of participants had insomnia or another serious sleep problem. With this setting the scene, Wiseman goes on to explain what happens when you don't get enough sleep – spoiler alert: nothing good.

"*Belenskys's study reveals the highly pernicious nature of even a small amount of sleep deprivation. Just a few nights sleeping for seven hours or less and your brain goes into slow motion. To make matters worse you will continue to feel fine and so don't make allowances for your sluggish mind. Within just a couple of days this level of sleep deprivation transforms you into an accident waiting to happen.*" (P67)

Dr Jacob Teitelbaum says the defining way to separate Fibromyalgia from any other cause of widespread pain and fatigue is to ask how well they sleep. If a patient sleeps with no trouble, according to Teitelbaum, they don't have Fibromyalgia. His SHINE protocol puts sleep at the beginning of the treatment. Without sleep, we can't get better. I agree. Teitelbaum's book *From Fatigued to Fantastic (2021)* is one of my top books about fibromyalgia, and his treatment approach gels with everything I have experienced. Without the sleep LDN was able to give me, I would never have begun to experience improvements. Though I do wonder what 'better' means for the large percentages of people in his studies that are lots better or better after the SHINE protocol. For me, my quality of life is currently hugely improved, but I still have a chronic illness that impacts me all day, every day. We might have different definitions of improvement.

Insomnia is:

A key problem for people with fibromyalgia and many other chronic illnesses

Debilitating and makes other already incapacitating symptoms worse

A recipe for a shorter, less fulfilled life

Pain inducing even for those without chronic pain conditions

A money drain in health care costs from those who suffer the side effects, in absenteeism from inability to work, and in lost income. If you could place a value on a fully functioning human being able to participate fully in life then multiply that by the 10 million people estimated in the US alone (and 3-6% of the world's population) it would be a massive number

And sleep:

Helps pretty much every symptom of fibromyalgia

Improves our quality of life and our emotional state

We can improve our sleep. It might be multifactorial, and a doctor needs to help in many cases, but we can improve sleep.

Taking Sleep Seriously

Does anyone else find it ridiculous that many millions of people are exhausted, struggling to get to sleep, to stay asleep, to wake feeling refreshed, to have sufficient energy to live; yet their doctors are not generally working their butts off to help find a solution?

After ten years battling Fibromyalgia mostly alone, I was referred to a pain specialist at the hospital, and she dismissed my sleep problems, saying medicine won't help, and I should try some more sleep hygiene. Now, I go to bed around the same time every day, don't have caffeine after lunch, take my time to wind down, do a body scan meditation before going to sleep, partake in gentle exercise most days, and so on. I have also tried chamomile tea, Sleep Drops, 5-HTP, melatonin, and magnesium, and I had been on amitriptyline for around 10 years at the time. I have done all these things for a long time. I wouldn't have been begging for help or looking into medicine if anything had worked.

I have always known that sleep makes a massive difference for me. If I can spend nine hours in bed to achieve eight hours of broken sleep, I feel so much better.

Going back to Dr Jacob Teitelbaum, MD, and Dr Genevra Liptan, MD, these two prominent physicians with Fibromyalgia write about how to recover. They both state that sleep is the basis for recovery. They recommend both natural and pharmaceutical options, and they acknowledge how important sleep is to getting well.

I have come a long way. I have implemented an entire lifestyle change, including reduced work hours, supplementation, gentle exercise, meditation, and rest. But I couldn't get any further without help with my sleep.

This is where Low Dose Naltrexone (LDN) comes in. You can learn more about LDN in my chapter dedicated to it. Essentially this medicine finally helped me to sleep in more than one-hour blocks. The flow on effect of this has improved the quality of my life dramatically. Not fighting so hard for sleep, achieving sleep cycles, and getting proper sleep has made as big a difference as I hypothesized it would.

Dr David Hanscom estimates in his book *Back in Control: A Surgeon's Journey Out of Chronic Pain* that 40% of people with insomnia developed chronic pain. In my experience, my number one recommendation to anyone suffering from chronic pain or similar illnesses is to get your sleep.

Don't be fobbed off here. This is an area for you to continually work on. Even with everything I know and do, I struggle to get enough sleep and to achieve deep sleep.

Things That Can Help

Sleep hygiene is something you will probably hear about at some point. It is a set of tips that can make getting to sleep easier. There are a lot of options, so you must create a sleep hygiene routine that works for you.

Here are some basic sleep hygiene tips that I follow:

- Don't have caffeine after lunch
- Have a wind-down routine that doesn't involve technology
- Go to bed and get up at approximately the same time each day
- Expose yourself to sunlight early in the day
- Adjust your bed to your needs (i.e., suitable mattress, mattress topper, the right pillow, weather-suitable

blankets)

- Eat a small protein-based snack before bed
- Have a warm bath with Epsom salts
- Apply magnesium oil
- Manage the pain as best as you can
- Dab lavender oil on temples and wrists
- Use your heat pack. (I love my electric heating pad and use it at bedtime and throughout the night.)
- Do a body scan meditation or a full Yoga Nidra meditation. (I do one right before I go to sleep and again if I wake in the night.)

Here are some natural sleep aids you can try:

- Revitalizing Sleep Formula (an all-in-one herbal mix)
- Other formulas with the herbal sleep remedies such as Valerian root
- Lemon balm
- GABA supplement
- Chamomile tea
- 5-HTP
- Essential oils
- Melatonin
- CBD oil

Other sleep aids:

- Amitriptyline or another prescribed antidepressant for the sedating effect. (I took it for over a decade and finally was able to come off it once the LDN was helping.)
- Over the counter medicines to help with sleep

- Pain relief (Part of my sleep woes is due to neck pain. Prior to bed I take a dose of pain medicine, if needed, to help get a jump start on the night.).
- Temporary use of prescribed sleep aids as prescribed and monitored by your doctor

You may find the template on the next page useful for tracking your sleep and any sleep hygiene methods you enact. It is available to download on my website.

My Mindful Evening routine

I recommend creating a mindful evening routine that you can maintain most nights to help cue your body for sleep. You could include a gentle self-massage, warm bath, gentle stretches, restorative yoga, breathing practice, meditation, reading, a warming cup of non-caffeinated tea (if going to the bathroom overnight isn't a problem for you), gratitude practice, and more.

How my mindful bedtime routine looks:

Take supplements and medicines at 9pm

Begin wind down routine including hygiene like washing face and brushing teeth

Gentle stretches

Read something low key in bed with my electric heating pad

Legs on cushion restorative yoga pose

Body scan meditation

This is what I do most nights. Sometimes I cut out bits and pieces of it, but the framework is the same.

Action Points

- Start tracking your sleep with a sleep diary
- Write a list of what you already do
- Write a list of what you would like to try and discuss with your doctor

Start trying things! I highly recommend doing a Yoga Nidra guided meditation before bed as a first line of defence. This will help with so many things beyond sleep but is proven to help you get to sleep. Find a free Yoga Nidra download for yourself at https://www.melissavsfibromyalgia.com/book-goodie-bag/

Sleep Diary

Date	Hours	Supplements/Medicines

Central Sensitivity/ Overactive Nervous System

As we looked at earlier, the central nervous system is a big factor in fibromyalgia. Trauma of all kinds can trip our nervous system into overdrive. A lot of research suggests that Fibromyalgia is the result of central nervous system dysfunction – specifically an overactive nervous system, stressing and exhausting the brain (Dennis W. Dobritt, *Fibromyalgia – A Brief Overview*)[16]. Other literature suggests that chronic pain causes the central nervous system to go into overdrive. However you look at it, the nervous system appears to be involved.

The theory of autonomic nervous system dysfunction resonates with me as a big part of the puzzle, but it is not the entire answer.

A lot of programmes are popping up claiming to "cure" chronic pain. (Lightning Process, Curable app, the CFS Unravelled programme, and various books with similar programmes.) This is based upon the idea of retraining the brain. If these programmes are the entire answer for someone, I

[16] Dennis W. Dobritt, DO, DABPM, FIPP. *Fibromyalgia - A Brief Overview (a presentation)*. Retrieved from
www.michigan.gov/documents/mdch/fibroacpsm_246421_7.pdf

am happy for them. But mostly they are going to be one part of the puzzle.

Recently, I read Dr David Hanscom's book *Back in Control*, which outlines his programme for recovery from chronic pain[17]. It is heavily based upon rewiring the brain, but he also includes several other key components, including sleep. He emphasizes how important sleep is and believes that before a person can be successful with treating chronic pain, they must be sleeping well. I don't agree with all his ideas, but I do like the fact that he recognizes the multiple components that are part of chronic pain-based illnesses. It is worth a read.

There are theories of anxiety and depression causing, or being the result of, Fibromyalgia. However, it is normal for people with constant pain, fatigue and other symptoms who are gaslighted by everyone in their lives, particularly medical professionals, to feel sad and to appear depressed (lethargy from extreme fatigue, for example). Depression and anxiety are just other parts of the puzzle for a lot of us. I believe they are an effect, rather than the cause.

One of the key things I learnt from the first pain specialist I saw was about central sensitization. He helped me to see that by not treating my pain appropriately, I was causing more pain. (I had a thing about avoiding medicines and trying to take as little as possible.) I was changing physiologically as a response to the ongoing pain and causing my nervous system to go into overdrive. So, in addition to treating my pain, I needed to calm

---

[17] Dr David Hansom, MD. 2016. Back in Control. Vertus Press.

my nervous system down.

Luckily for me, prior to learning about this theory, I had already laid the groundwork and made great progress with my overactive nervous system. Through meditation, which I have been practicing for years now, I no longer react as strongly to things that would have made my heart pound, breathing quicken, and have me looking for the exit. Things that used to make me anxious no longer do. I also have the tools to calm myself down when my nervous system does go into overdrive. If I notice that I am getting wound up and my heart rate is climbing rapidly, I will quietly take several deep, gentle breaths, immediately calming my system. When I am feeling overwhelmed overall, I will sneak away to my room and meditate.

Meditation and mindfulness are great ways to help train your brain to calm down. Dr. Hanscom also recommends free writing once or twice a day for five or ten minutes and then ripping up the page as a way of creating separation from issues. Some might also benefit from counselling or specific work on trauma-induced anxiety. We talk more about meditation later in the book as this is my preferred method of helping calm the central nervous system while getting good rest at the same time.

Hypothalamic Dysfunction

I had been grasping at the ends of some complex strands of answers for a while when I came upon a new term, "hypothalamic dysfunction". It was like a light shone down and angels sang Hallelujah. As I read, I was nodding my head and making connections.

When I came upon the term "Hypothalamic-pituitary-adrenal axis dysfunction" so many things clicked into place. There was a list of symptoms that I had not only conquered and forgot I had, but the rest of my symptoms were also there.

All the disparate suggestions that get thrown at people with Fibromyalgia made sense. The problem was that they were too far down the line. For example, one common suggestion is recommending a specific supplement for supporting the adrenal glands. Yes, the adrenal glands may need help, but a random supplement without working on the higher stream effects is too far removed.

The brain is the boss.

While the brain may be the boss, it is not in the way many people write fibromyalgia off - as all in the head, needing antidepressants and therapy. Although those could be useful complementary therapies. Actual physiological changes occur in the brain which causes a domino effect downstream to all the key systems. Immune, hormone, digestion etc. Affecting pain processing, sleep, memory, cognition, etc.

There are far smarter people without cognitive impairment who write about this stuff, so I will let you Google those keywords above for more detail.

The point is that looking back enabled me to realise that I had accidentally stumbled upon keys to my dramatic improvement. Looking for a supplement here or there isn't enough. It takes a complex, whole of life protocol:

- Managing neuroinflammation (with low dose naltrexone)
- Helping the mitochondria get fuel (with Recovery Factors supplement)
- Reducing perpetuating factors (reducing work and computer time, decreasing stressors)
- Good nutrition (supporting gut health, energy and removing more perpetuating factors)
- Calming the central nervous system (with yoga, meditation and breathing)
- Physiotherapy and gentle dry needling to help with the trigger points (reducing the pain, reduces inflammation and fatigue)

I had halved my pain and fatigue levels, improved my sleep, increased my quality of life, balanced my blood sugar levels (hypoglycaemic-like reactions), and more. But there was more to do. I still didn't manage enough deep sleep, needed a rest each afternoon, managed pain at all times, and basically lived a reduced life. It was emotionally bolstering to find these threads to follow but I knew that my journey would be continuing for a while yet.

Action Points

If you haven't downloaded the free Yoga Nidra guided meditation, please scan the code below, and try it every night before bed or each day as a rest.

BOOK GOODIE BAG

Low Dose Naltrexone: The Medicine That Has Changed My Life

Medicines are a tricky business when it comes to Fibromyalgia. What works for one may not work for another. In addition, side effects are generally noticeable and often the effects of the drug wear off after time.

Low dose Naltrexone (LDN) has been such an amazing find for me. Being able to achieve better sleep and all the positive offshoots of that is something I am grateful for every single day.

About LDN

Naltrexone is an opioid antagonist that works differently in the body when taken at a lower dose. Usually prescribed for alcohol and opioid addictions at doses of 50mg or more, low dose Naltrexone is usually anything from .25mg – 6mg. LDN works in the endocannabinoid system. It temporarily blocks the receptors encouraging the body to make more endorphins. There is research suggesting that a cause of Fibromyalgia could be due to an endocannabinoid deficiency.[18] Given how well it

---

[18] Ethan B. Russo. 2016. *Clinical Endocannabinoid Deficiency Reconsidered: Current Research Supports the Theory in Migraine, Fibromyalgia, Irritable*

helps me, it could be a plausible explanation.

However Fibromyalgia may originate, I like the fact that LDN essentially spurs your own body into action and that there are few side effects. There is also plenty of research and patient evidence. I believe that patient-evidence. his term, which I love, was coined by Julia Schopick in her book *Honest Medicine*. It's a very important term. That's your voice, not the researcher's voice.

An interesting thing about LDN is that different doses help different people, and it can take widely varied amounts of time to work. These research studies currently taking place (as below) using a standard dose of 4.5mg for about eight weeks are not going to give us the full picture. They are a great start, however.

It can take some time to see the benefits, though most of the trials start patients at 4.5mg immediately and last around eight weeks. In practice, for myself and for people in the LDN groups I am in, we tend to need to start our doses lower and titrate up (increase our dose) slowly.

Side effects, such as insomnia, headache, and vivid dreams, are generally short-lived and limited. Then compare this to the usually prescribed fibromyalgia medicines which can cause worse symptoms than they are meant to help manage. Which seems like the better option? Also, LDN causes no withdrawal symptoms other than your body suffering because it was making a difference. You don't need to reduce your dose. When I went off LDN prior to having my third baby there were

Bowel, and Other Treatment-Resistant Syndromes. 1(1): 154–165. doi: 10.1089/can.2016.0009.

absolutely no withdrawals or negative effects.

Research by Dr Jarred Younger has also been promising. Younger, along with Luke Parkitny and David McLain, started with a tiny study and found positive results; approximately 65% of patients have experienced clinically significant results[19]. In 2022, Dr Jarred Younger was involved with a bigger study, and early results sound promising. I look forward to the final paper[20].

I have seen many testimonies from people with Fibromyalgia experiencing changes due to LDN ranging from mildly beneficial to miraculous. There are also those for whom it does not work, or they do not try it for long enough. This is not a quick fix for most patients

Further information on how LDN works is well-explained by Dr Jill Carnahan, MD, in her article *Low Dose Naltrexone: The New Treatment You've Never Heard* Of on her website[21], which includes many links to research.

Low dose naltrexone came on my radar in 2016, and after consuming all the research and anecdotal evidence about its impact on Fibromyalgia, I earmarked it for my major experiment after I had my baby. I had my baby in December 2016 and nursed until April 2017. I began LDN after that.

---

[19] Jarred Younger, Luke Parkitny, & David McLain, *The Use of Low-Dose Naltrexone (LDN) as a Novel Anti-Inflammatory Treatment for Chronic Pain* (2014), retrieved from ncbi.nlm.nih.gov/pmc

[20] UAB, College of Arts and Science. (n.d.) Current Projects. Retrieved from https://cas.uab.edu/

[21] Found here https://www.jillcarnahan.com/2015/12/19/low-dose-naltrexone-the-treatment-youve-never-heard-of/

LDN and Pregnancy –
An Area to Research Carefully

I learned afterward that it is potentially safe to take LDN until the 37th week. I believe this is because you generally go into labour anytime from 37-42 weeks and you may need opioids during the labour. Though it appears unlikely to have been a problem. A pharmacist on the LDN Research Trust's website says, *"The half-life of Low Dose Naltrexone is about 4 hours. So, when it is taken there is a blockade that gradually reduces over the course of 4 hours to half the amount, and then again by half in the next 4 hours. At this point, it is probably not clinically relevant."*[22] So, if one takes their dose an hour before bedtime, by the morning it should be clinically irrelevant.

There are fertility clinics that use LDN specifically to help women with autoimmune conditions to maintain a pregnancy. Therefore, there are a lot of women who have been given LDN for pregnancy. But this is a decision you and your doctor must make after looking at the available evidence, which includes anecdotal evidence as research into medicines during pregnancy would be unethical.

There are no long-term studies yet. As with all medicine used in pregnancy, it would be a matter of balancing cost versus benefits. Would LDN help more than the potential risks? I did

[22] How Long Does Low Dose Naltrexone Take to Block the Body's Receptors https://ldnresearchtrust.org/how-long-does-low-dose-naltrexone-ldn-take-block-body%E2%80%99s-receptors

this in conjunction with my doctor and a specialist for amitriptyline for all my pregnancies. We concluded that I was already sleeping so poorly due to pregnancy that coming off it would only add to more stress on my body.

Dr Phil Boyle presents his findings in a presentation called Low Dose Naltrexone in Pregnancy (n.d.). He shows the comparison of outcomes between those in his clinic that used LDN and those that didn't, and the results were positive. On the flipside of that, a study on animals using LDN during pregnancy was not-so-positive, as documented on the LDN Now website.

It is considered potentially safe for breastfeeding – this is discussed on Drugs.com in the article *Naltrexone Use While Breasting* (n.d.):

"Limited data indicate that naltrexone is minimally excreted into breast milk. If naltrexone is required by the mother, it is not a reason to discontinue breastfeeding."

Please note: This is a finding on the usual dose of Naltrexone, often used to help detox off drugs.

My Experiment

I believed if I could experience a 30% decrease in pain and fatigue, my life would change. This is considered clinically significant and therefore a success. I could be a mama, a wife, do my work, have some form of a life outside of this, and not pay with such significant levels of pain, fatigue, and other side effects of Fibromyalgia.

I can only share research and what works or doesn't work

for me. As I've mentioned before, we are all unique and react differently. If you're interested in learning more about LDN after reading this book,, please read the research and information, and then discuss it with your doctor.

I began LDN in April 2017. I had a small baby who had reflux and didn't sleep well, so it was a trial by fire for LDN. I began on 0.5mg and titrated up slowly. Side effects included vivid dreams for the first few nights at a new dose. I also experienced a surge of ulcers and cold sores in the beginning of my treatment. I believe this was my immune system coming back online appropriately.

The effects were subtle. After a few months, I accidentally skipped two nights close to each other and found myself feeling like I was hit by a truck carrying a whopping amount of fatigue.

After several months, I noted an increase in stamina, slightly decreased fatigue, and slightly decreased neck pain. It was a challenge to note because the second I have more energy, I use it. I am my own worst enemy at times. My average pain levels went from around 4-7/10 down to 3-5/10 with higher levels being a flare up caused by ignoring my limits.

Without external interference, in the guise of, say, a cute squishy baby, the combination of amitriptyline and LDN appeared to help me sleep slightly better. I often attained blocks of sleep in a row, sometimes up to five or six hours. This almost never happened previously.

There are six main ways that LDN helps me:

Sleep

First and foremost is sleep. For the ten years or so prior to LDN, I had not slept in more than one-hour blocks, that's rarely completing a whole sleep cycle, therefore my body was in chronic deep sleep deprivation. Since LDN, I can sleep in two, three, four or even five-hour blocks! I am so grateful for this; I can't even tell you. I believe this is what has created the other benefits.

Please do note that I still enact my sleep hygiene list daily (see the chapter on sleep).

Pain

Since around nine months into treatment, I have noticed a reduction in neck pain. Neck pain has been a constant problem over 10 years. In 2017, while starting LDN, I learnt that my neck issue is actually MPS. After throwing the severe, recurring muscle knots, also known as trigger points, into the fibro basket, I finally had an answer. The physiotherapist has been helping me to work on these trigger points through intramuscular needling by gently inserting a tiny needle into the trigger point and letting it relax a little. They also worked on neck mobilisations. This, and sleep, which potentially reduced my Fibromyalgia levels of pain and fatigue, have helped. My pain levels were 6-8/10 with severe headaches with daily dizziness and nausea in 2010 before I started this journey. Just prior to LDN they were approximately 4-6/10 with occasional severe headaches. In early 2018, after one year on LDN, the average was 3-4/10 with the occasional spike to 5/10 with a bad headache and was usually due to me overdoing things.

Emotional

If you haven't lived with pain that interrupts sleep, which interferes with life all day, every day for over a decade or been unable to sleep for more than an hour at a time, it would be hard to convey the depth of impact on my emotional well-being.

It was a huge and welcome change to not have to fight to sleep at 3am, and not swap pillows and apply heat or pain cream to try and induce sleep.

My quality of life is so much better. I never let myself lose hope, but it was dwindling. This was a necessary win.

Stamina

Slowly my stamina increased. I was able to tolerate activities that used to wipe me out. I can exercise a little bit longer. Overall, I can do a little more compared to my life before LDN. Having had a baby with reflux, I feel I coped exceptionally well and that is because of LDN.

Fatigue

Fatigue is the second of my two worst symptoms with neck pain being the first. Yes, that's *is* not was. My fatigue has improved but I still have a limited energy envelope. I can get through the day on a 15-minute meditation and a brief sit down with my heat pack. I still can't physically stay up past 10pm or out past 7pm and that's a fair trade off to me.

Immunity

Since I began LDN I have experienced a lot less illness. Viral flares of existing issues such as cold sores, which were rampant in the early months on LDN, are now few and far between. I get general illnesses like cold and flu far less frequently. I was sick all the time prior to the beginning of this wellness journey, and I caught almost everything my kids did prior to adding LDN to my life. This is quite a bonus.

Another interesting effect was that I lost weight. I was at my pre-Fibromyalgia weight prior to my third pregnancy and lost the weight easily after my fourth pregnancy.

LDN And My Third And Fourth Pregnancies

My third and fourth pregnancies were much better experiences, despite severe pelvis issues which impacted my mobility and caused high pain levels. Going into each pregnancy with a better baseline made each one easier to manage. I was also able to nurse beyond a year with both when previously I had trouble with supply. I went off LDN at 37 weeks because my first child came at 37 weeks and 4 days, and I wanted to be sure I was clear of the medication in case I needed an epidural and opioid medication. I resumed LDN as soon as I got home from the hospital.

Meditation: Multiple Birds With One Stone

Meditation is a fabulous tool for fibromyalgia/chronic pain/chronic fatigue. Anything that promotes deep rest is a helpful addition to our toolkit. Anyone following my work for any amount of time will know how much I love Yoga Nidra guided meditation.

Loads of us have heard the spiel: the idea that it will be a magical panacea. I get it. Many of us have tried meditation to little benefit. This happens specially when we have been told to try it seated either on a cushion or hard floor. I want my meditation to double as profound rest. And I want the secondary benefits. So let's talk about the benefits of meditation, the types you can do, and how you can build your own meditation practice.

Around 2015 I began practicing and, as I experienced the benefits, I started researching and learning more. This is an obvious fact that is illustrated on my blog which has more than 300 posts and, of course, I have authored several successful books. I am a questioner who loves research! I began to link the benefits of meditation to a deeper root cause of fibromyalgia. In the Fibromyalgia Framework Series, I linked meditation as a key tool for managing the central nervous system overdrive that exists in fibromyalgia.

As I mentioned previously in this book, fibromyalgia appears to be the result of an overactive nervous system. Specifically, hypothalamic dysfunction. Google *"hypothalamic dysfunction fibromyalgia"* and you get 12,500 results. Google *"neuroinflammation fibromyalgia"* and you get 212,000 results. Search *"central nervous system fibromyalgia"* and you get over two million results. There is something here! My brain-foggy brain hasn't got there yet; I just know this is the right direction.

Key point: It is part of the brain structure, not in your head. It is not psychosomatic. It cannot be fixed by counselling, although counselling may be a helpful part of healing because it is stressful and hard to live with constant pain, fatigue, insomnia, etc. I cannot state this enough.

Meditation helps calm the central nervous system.

Some people believe that the presence of chronic pain results in changes to the brain. Meditation can help reverse these changes. *"Through meditation, Dr. Pohl hopes to reverse some of the negative changes in the brain that can occur with chronic pain. "We have seen a decrease in cortisol and epinephrine levels, an increase in serotonin and gamma-aminobutyric acid levels, which are linked to relaxation and anti-depression, and an increase in natural killer cells. With sufficient practice, patients can establish patterns of thought that diminish catastrophization, thus decreasing pain,"he said."*[23]

---

[23] *Meditation: A Pathway to Pain* available on Practical Pain Management website

It's not simple though. You can't just "fix" the brain issue and be cured. Because the body is a whole – all our systems are connected. Doctor Rutherford of Power Health, who has several talks about fibromyalgia on his YouTube channel, considers the brain to be the first domino. There are downward effects that affect other systems of the body. Hence the complexity of our symptoms.

Plus, we don't have a way to magically fix the brain. Low dose Naltrexone can help with neuroinflammation. Calming the central nervous system can help. We have the tools to dramatically reduce our symptoms but not a cure.

So, what concrete steps can we take? We can investigate reducing neuroinflammation, manage the central nervous system, and work on the big dominoes. This is where meditation comes in.

Benefits Of Meditation For Fibromyalgia

- Complete rest
- Calming the central nervous system
- A break from stimulus
- Mindfulness - Focus on the body, accepting it as it is
- Not trying to nap, which can be frustrating for those who can't
- For those who have trouble with orthostatic intolerance, just lying down can make you feel better

- A boost in energy however temporary
- Improve the immune system (University Health News Daily, 2018)
- Treat depression
- Reduced anxiety
- Reduce pain

How Can You Meditate?

Breath focus: Simply focus on your breath for a few moments. Focus on how you breathe in and how the breath feels a little warmer on the way out. Notice how your body feels when you exhale. Observe how your breaths get a little longer as you relax. Don't push anything, just observe.

Do your own body scan meditation by quietly thinking of each part of your body in turn, noticing the feeling in each, accepting it, willing that part to relax and moving to the next.

Progressive relaxation: By tensing and releasing each part of your body in turn, you can encourage it to relax deeply. As an example, you could start with your feet, tense and release your lower legs, upper legs, glutes, abdomen, arms, and face.

Guided meditations: There are body scan meditations, Yoga Nidra, mindfulness meditations, and meditation specific to pain or fatigue, etc.

How do you experience the benefits of meditation? By doing it regularly. Make a commitment and practice.

I have meditated almost every day for several years. I cannot cope without it now because it provides deep rest after lunch to counteract the poor quality of sleep and the fatigue. It is fundamental to my pacing plan and my whole life management.

You need to find the type that resonates with you the most so that you will continue it.

I suggest Yoga Nidra guided meditation because you can do it lying down and in your bed with your heat pack. It's perfect for people with chronic pain and fatigue!

You can do it:

- First thing in the morning if you don't feel you've slept well
- During a flare
- In place of a rest/nap. It's especially useful if you cannot nap but really wish you could.
- After work
- Before bed
- During the night. It's great for those painsomnia nights
- Basically, whenever suits you

The thing about Yoga Nidra or any meditation is that it should feel good in the moment and give you some much needed rest. But it is also quietly working in the long term. Let's delve deeper into Yoga Nidra in the next chapter.

Meditation Guidance/Scripts

Breath-focus

Simply focus on your breath for a few moments wherever you are, whenever you need.

Get comfortable, however that looks for you where you are.

Breathe normally a few times.

Send your attention to your breath now.

Notice how you breathe in. That the breath feels a little warmer on the way out. How your body feels when you exhale. How your breaths get a little longer as you relax.

Don't push anything, just observe for as long as is comfortable.

Body Scan Meditation

You can do this anywhere, anytime. It is a great practice for relaxing into rest or sleep.

Get comfortable, wherever you are right now.

Take a few gentle breaths. Notice how you feel right now.

Bring your attention to your right hand, noticing the feeling in your right hand. The thumb and each finger. The palm and back of the hand. Bathe it in your attention. Invite it to relax.

Move your attention, mindfully, to your right arm. Noticing your whole right arm. Invite it to relax.

When you're ready, slide your attention to your right shoulder, right side of chest and waist.

Right leg. Pay attention to your whole right leg. Invite each part of it to relax. Paying special attention to the parts that draw your notice.

Bring your attention to your right foot. All of the toes. The top and sole of the foot. Invite it to relax.

Bring your attention to your left hand, noticing the feeling in your left hand. The thumb and each finger. The palm and back of the hand. Bathe it in your attention. Invite it to relax.

Move your attention, mindfully, to your left arm. Noticing your whole left arm. Invite it to relax.

When you're ready, slide your attention to your left shoulder, left side of chest and waist.

left leg. Pay attention to your whole left leg. Invite each part of it to relax. Paying special attention to the parts that draw your attention.

Bring your attention to your left foot and all your toes. Observe the top and sole of the foot. Invite it to relax.

Let your attention encompass both of your feet. Both legs. Lower back. Middle back. Upper back. Both shoulders. Back of the neck. Left side of the neck, right side of the neck. Base of the skull. Invite the base of the skull to relax. Back of the head. Top of the head. Forehead. Right eye, left eye. Right temple, left temple. Nose. Right cheek, left cheek. Jaw. Tongue. Throat. Chest. Abdomen. Pelvis.

Notice your whole body. Invite your whole body to relax. Take several, gentle, deep breaths and stay like this for as long as is comfortable.

My Favourite Tool Ever: Yoga Nidra Guided Meditation

Yoga Nidra is also known as "yogic sleep". The brain waves during Yoga Nidra mimic those in sleep. For some of us, it is the only way to reach the deepest stages of restorative sleep. There is a common belief that a session feels like three hours of sleep.

Yoga Nidra is like meditation, but in some way, it's not. Some parts of meditation are included in Yoga Nidra. But Nidra has a specific sequence. It begins with grounding into the moment by focusing on sounds and our breath). Setting an intention (or san kalpa) is an important part of it. This is a positive, present tense focus that you usually use until you see fruition. You then move through a body scan. Spend time witnessing thoughts and playing with the sensation of opposites. There is a period near the end where you are able to rest in the moment. This is my favourite part. Often by this point, I am so relaxed that I am able to enjoy a quiet body with limited sensations which is a relief for someone with a loud body at all other times. At this point, for experienced meditators, it can feel like you have drifted off to sleep. If you wake as soon as the teacher guides you out, then you were not asleep, but were in deep meditation.

An important note here is that most teachers will ask you to set the intention to stay awake and aware. However, I believe the biggest benefit Yoga Nidra offers us is the chance for some deep rest. If you can catch a nap at this time, take it.

As I mentioned earlier, a theory about Fibromyalgia is that the sympathetic nervous system, also known as our fight-or-flight response, may be stuck in overdrive. Meditation promotes a calming of this system, allowing the parasympathetic nervous system to activate. Yoga Nidra takes the benefits of "normal" meditation a step further with its sequencing and movement through brainwave patterns.

Yoga Nidra offers the following benefits:

- Helps with chronic insomnia
- Calms the central nervous system
- Can improve the immune system
- May help with depression and anxiety
- Reduces pain and fatigue
- Relieves stress

After a 20-minute session, my pain levels can drop to as low as 3/10 and decrease my fatigue levels to a similar place. The effects help me get through the busy evening period with my kids. Without this proper rest break, the afternoon does not feel good. I feel lethargic, exhausted and like I need about five hours of sleep.

It's not easy to carve out these uninterrupted minutes. However, it is such an important tool for management that I prioritise it as much as possible.

Kamini Desai PHD, in her book *Yoga Nidra: The Art of Transformational Sleep* (2017) describes Yoga Nidra as being used as a nap and says that *"Using Yoga Nidra as a nap is like using a jet plane to drive to the grocery store. You can do it, but it is a gross under-utilization of its potential."* (p7) This book talks a lot about using Yoga Nidra to initiate the relaxation response and its positive effects on our bodies. It helps us to reset our overactive nervous system. In the section on the benefits Yoga Nidra has for us, Desai refers specifically to fibromyalgia:

"Yoga Nidra as meditation increases the brain's production of serotonin... Low serotonin can be related to depression, anxiety, bipolar disorder, apathy, low self-esteem, obesity, insomnia, migraine headaches, premenstrual syndrome, and fibromyalgia." (p.209)

How many people with our syndromes don't have at least two on the above-mentioned list?

This paper from 2020 on the effectiveness of Yoga Nidra states: *"Empirical studies on Yoga Nidra confirm positive effects on various physiological and psychological criteria such as insomnia, addictive behavior, chronic diseases, pain therapy, pregnancies, geriatrics, asthma as well as disorders of the cardiovascular system (e.g., Satyananda Saraswati 2009). Not only based on self-reports, but also by imaging techniques such as positron emission tomography (PET) and electroencephalography (EEG), sustained changes in the activation of the brain were recorded (e.g., Lou et al. 1999; Mandlik et al. 2002;)."*[24]

Research is still limited, but it is bearing out my experience.

[24] Moszeik, E.N., von Oertzen, T. & Renner, KH. Effectiveness of a short Yoga Nidra meditation on stress, sleep, and well-being in a large and diverse sample.

Yoga Nidra and Me

It took me a while to appreciate meditation. It was years, in fact, for me to consider giving up precious reading time for it. When I first started improving, I was so happy to be able to read, which meant it was hard to give up.

In 2014, I read a book about mindfulness meditation and found a YouTube video of a Yoga Nidra session called *Yoga Nidra - Deeply Restorative Guided Relaxation/Meditation* that I particularly liked. I avoided the spiritual and religious aspects of it. Once I watched that video, it was off to the races to give it a try. I am not sure what made me choose Yoga Nidra as opposed to the many other wonderful meditations on YouTube, but I am forever thankful I did.

I have meditations, body scans and Yoga Nidra of varying lengths that I like to switch between depending on my mood and wellbeing on any given day. I also use the body scan technique most nights to relax into sleep. The focus on the breath is like second nature to fall into. Now, when I am stuck awake in the middle of the night, usually after the kids have woken me, instead of tossing and turning in frustration, I do a body scan meditation. Not stressing about not sleeping combined with the effects of the deep rest are both restorative and usually lead back to sleep.

When I was pregnant and desperately tired and sore, meditation made a huge difference to my quality of life.

Sometimes, I would catch 5-10 minutes of sleep after the meditation finished and feel uniquely restored. On days when I have not slept well, it is deeply soothing to be able to rest completely without wishing I could nap.

The benefits of meditation have pervaded all facets of my life. I no longer get anxious without due cause. I feel profoundly calmed by the fact that I can attain deep rest in the face of constant fatigue and chronic insomnia, and I adore that this coping mechanism is freely available to me any time, any place.

I love meditation so much that in 2021 I completed my 200-hour Certified Meditation Teacher program in addition to a few Yoga Nidra specific training completed earlier in 2020. It's become my dream and my pleasure to share the tools that meditation and yoga offer to others who need some good rest too.

Yoga Nidra is also one of the first things I suggest when mentoring other people with chronic illness. It doesn't require energy, mobility or to be flare-free. In fact, it will likely help with all three.

Action Points

Did you download the free Yoga Nidra guided meditation from earlier? If not, scan the code below to do that. Try it every night before bed or each day as a rest.

I have an entire program dedicated to using Yoga Nidra for Chronic Pain and Fatigue. There is a link on the page above for you.

BOOK GOODIE BAG

Yoga For Fibromyalgia: It's Not What You Think

Yoga has become a bone of contention in the chronic illness world. This is for two reasons. One, people are touting it as a cure all. As much as yoga can help, it is only ONE part of my whole of life wellness plan. This has turned a lot of people with chronic illness off from trying it. And two, the idea of what yoga is thanks to some Instagram ideals and studio norms of what practice looks like. So, before we delve into how yoga helps me and my experience, let me start by saying that it is not about the length of your classes, how flexible one is, and there is more than just the physical practice. It is far more adaptable than people realise. Fun fact: Yoga asana postures were created to help yogis sit longer and more comfortably for meditation.

I am a yoga teacher who has practiced for more than a decade and I have never done a 90-minute class. In fact, most of my classes are around 15 or 20 minutes and that includes the savasana (final relaxation pose). Fun fact number two: Restorative yoga is a profoundly restful type of yoga that was designed specifically for those who are injured or unwell. As a yoga teacher I create classes for specific purposes, but the overarching goal of my personal practice and what I share with students is calming the central nervous system. Fun fact number three: I talk about yoga as tools for us and those tools fit right into our symptom management plans.

Check out my free Yoga for Chronic Pain and Fatigue series for samples of each of the four tools. You can find it on my website.

My Yoga Journey

After years of wanting to do yoga but being frustrated at being unable to find appropriate classes, I had a yoga teacher come to my home and help me create a modified sequence. I used that sequence, in a few variations for better days or harder days, for years.

For the first several years of sharing my journey on my blog, I struggled with sharing resources. I recommended it to help people start practicing yoga with chronic pain and fatigue, but realized there was a gap in sharing resources, and so I decided to create those resources to fill this gap. I completed my 200-hour Certified Yoga Teacher Training program in 2019 and began creating those resources myself.

During my training I experimented with the entire journey of every pose working to create a repertoire of accessible yoga. The constant practice reduced my pain and fatigue levels, and I was in the best physical shape of my life. In training to share yoga tools with others, I have first helped myself.

Perhaps the most surprising finding was that the most useful benefit yoga offers, in my opinion, is rest. My work is about using yoga to get some decent rest and balance the central nervous system. The four classes I share in my free Yoga for Chronic Pain and Fatigue series which is available through my blog are: breathing, restorative yoga, gentle stretching practice, and Yoga Nidra guided meditation. The stretching class can be done fully seated.

The list of poses I don't do is longer than what I do. Due to severe pelvis issues that developed during my pregnancies, I cannot practice hip openers, forward flexion or create an uneven balance between my left and right legs. I don't do arm balances because it is hard on my upper back with a lot of active trigger points, and I don't do many inversions. I happily take those poses that do work for me and utilise them. I take the tools yoga offers and use them in my daily symptom management plans.

After more than a decade of learning to live well with Fibromyalgia, perhaps the most valuable learning I possess is the ability to tune in to my body. I am constantly analysing what works, what doesn't, what's causing what pain, and what helps which body parts. I have brought this into my yoga journey, which has had ebbs and flows over the amount of time I've dealt with the pain.

The value of yoga for a body with pain and fatigue can be found in:

The awareness of what you are doing with your body in each pose, consciously engaging the correct muscles and taking the correct stretch or benefit on offer.

The basis of the breath: Breathing is key to yoga and to

accessing the parasympathetic nervous system[25]. Even stretches encourage full use of the breath which offer relaxation benefits.

The invitation to be outside of usual mind chatter: It's so easy to be lost in the movement, the breath, and the experience of the pose.

The gentle strengthening: This is a favoured pose. Downward Facing Dog utilises all the key muscle groups.

The ease of fitting practice in: Some days, it can be 20 minutes on the mat and engaged in a flowing sequence. Others, it can be a few key stretches in snippets of minutes. And still on other days it can be one restorative pose for 10 minutes. Corpse pose can be used when sleep is being elusive, with or without a body scan relaxation. Yoga is adaptable to each and every person.

The practice of yoga also includes many options and I make use of the tools it offers. And some of these yoga tools include:

- Sequences focused on strengthening – I do a modified sun salutation sequence with additions when I feel I can.
- Stretching poses – You can see several on my YouTube channel.
- Yoga on your bed or chair
- Restorative sequences or one-off poses
- Yoga Nidra, guided meditation "yogic sleep" (see my chapter on Yoga Nidra)
- Yogic breathing

Yoga Nidra is especially healing for me. My ideal yoga

---

[25] Joe Miller. (n.d.). *The Benefits of Yoga on the Parasympathetic Nervous System*. The Nest. Retrieved from the website http://woman.thenest.com.

practice would look like this: modified sun salutations first thing, gentle yogic stretches at work, Yoga Nidra after work, and legs on the chair pose in the evening. I never do all of this in one day, but one or two is great. Perhaps one of the best parts of yoga for Fibromyalgia is that you can fine tune it to your experience, your day, and your mood. If the fatigue is bad and post-exertional malaise has been plaguing you, you can choose a few poses and take breaks. If a particular body part has been upset, you can gently stretch all the muscles around it to free it up. If you're desperate for a break from your mind and its constant noise, you can do a guided Yoga Nidra session and let the voice take over for a time. Final fun fact about yoga: If I were only ever allowed to teach and use one yoga tool, it would be Yoga Nidra. You can do it in bed with your heat pack; it allows us profound rest and relaxation which is difficult to get any other way, and helps us with so many other functions. This is likely contrary to what you imagined when you thought of "yoga" before.

Research

Type "yoga for fibromyalgia" or "yoga for myofascial pain syndrome" or "yoga for pain" etc., and you will find a wealth of search options to delve into.

There is research specifically for using poses for myofascial pain syndrome, fibromyalgia, and more. Taking a more macroscopic view, mindfulness for chronic illness is just as much of a buzz topic at the moment with plenty of research supporting the benefits of mindfulness on chronic pain, fatigue, anxiety and more.

Take this 2010 study that found, "*pain was reduced in the yoga group by an average of 24 percent, fatigue by 30 percent and depression by 42 percent.*"[26] The yoga group participated in a holistic program for eight weeks, including gentle yoga poses, meditation, breathing exercises, yoga-based coping instructions, group discussions, and a daily diary assessing their progress. The control group received standard medication treatments.

This was followed up three months later: "*Follow-up results showed that patients sustained most of their post treatment gains, with the FIQR (Fibromyalgia Impact Questionnaire Revised) Total Score remaining 21.9% improved at 3 months. Yoga practice rates were good, and more practice was associated with more benefit for a variety of outcomes.*"[27]

This study was small, just eight participants completed the study on the effect of yoga on myofascial pain syndrome in the neck. It comprised two weeks of breathing and relaxation practices and two weeks of asanas (poses), breathing and relaxation. The poses were Trikonasan (triangle pose), Tadasan (mountain pose), Vakrasan (twisted pose), Balasan (child's pose) and Vajrasan (thunderbolt pose).

The results were that this program "*led to significant improvement in the quality of health, physical capacity (strength), cervical range of motion, and pressure threshold of the trigger*

[26] *A pilot randomized controlled trial of the Yoga of Awareness program in the management of fibromyalgia by J. W. Carson et al*

[27] *Follow-up of yoga of awareness for fibromyalgia: results at 3 months and replication in the wait-list group by J. W. Carson et al*

points, and decreased the disability and pain."[28]

Perspectives on Yoga Inputs in the Management of Chronic Pain

Describes the benefits: *"This consists of decreased metabolism,[24] decreased rate of breathing, decreased blood pressure, decreased muscle tension, decreased heart rate and increased slow brain [alpha] waves.[25] As the neural discharge pattern gets corrected, the habitual deep muscle hypertonicity and thus the static load on postural muscle also slowly come down. The function of viscera improves with the sense of relaxation and sleep gets deeper and sustained. The fatigue level comes down."[29]*

In summary, the benefits of yoga for chronic illness (or anyone):

- Calms the autonomic nervous system
- Help with sleep
- Reduced fatigue
- Reduced pain
- Increased physical capacity
- Decreased myofascial pain
- Less anxiety
- Reduced depression
- Relaxation
- Mindfulness of movement
- Awareness of proper alignment

What I love the most about yoga for managing chronic pain and fatigue is the ease of adapting it to my current abilities.

[28] *Effect of yoga on the Myofascial Pain Syndrome of neck by D Sharan et al*
[29] Perspectives on Yoga Inputs in the Management of Chronic Pain by Nandini Vallath Retrieved from the website http://woman.thenest.com.

102

Whatever my symptom level is any given day there is an option for me to practice yoga.

Let's talk a couple of key things here: Yoga is a tool, a multi-use tool, but a tool nonetheless. I will use any tool at my disposal to help with the symptoms I live with. In much the same way I use low dose Naltrexone because it was not designed for fibromyalgia or myofascial pain syndrome.

If some parts of the spectrum of yoga practices don't resonate with you, ignore them. If you want to look at it as a purely physical practice, then do so.

Examples of how yoga tools can help us in our journey:

Yoga helps with our pacing and as rest breaks, both brief and full. Yoga Nidra guided meditation is my big rest break, and I wouldn't function as well without it. We can also use breathing breaks, body scan meditations, one-off restorative poses (such as seated supported child's pose), and other poses for short rest stops in the day.

Next time you're at the office and need a stretching break you could try the following sequence:

Short day yoga break

Take a seated mountain pose, close your eyes, or let your gaze soften at a point in the distance. Take several deep breaths.

When you're ready, move into the following stretches:

Neck stretches. Exhale on the stretch, inhale when returning to the centre. Use micromovements here if needed, tip the head one inch in each direction.

Shoulder shrugs and circles

Raise your arms to a **tall mountain**. Clasp one hand over the other wrist and gently stretch to each side (swaying mountain). Keep the movement small, keep your torso upright (don't sink forward) and breathe into it. Hold for a few breaths on each side.

Lift one leg at a time and perform **toe points with calf stretches**. Hold for a few breaths each.

Sit tall and move into **seated cat and cow pose**. (Curve and arch your back). Allow as little or as much movement of the spine as is comfortable. Move with the breath.

Bring **one knee into the chest.** Hold here if comfortable or pull the knee over the opposite knee as far as is comfortable. Feel the stretch in your gluteus region and hold. Breathe deeply for as long as it feels good.

Stack your arms on the desk or table in front of you and lean forward for a **supported seated child's pose.** You may like to stack your fists one on top of the other and place your forehead on them if it is hard to reach the desk. Notice how it feels when you inhale and exhale. Pay attention to the sensations. Encourage your body to relax. Stay here as long as it is comfortable.

Stress management

Whenever you feel stress or anxiety rising, simply stop and take some deep breaths.

Inhale smoothly for a count of four, pause for two, exhale for six. Don't push it. You just want the exhale to be slightly longer than the inhale. Do this for as long as you like.

The above Short Day Yoga Break will also help with this. A body scan meditation, or restorative yoga pose will also help with this. Build a nest of several bolsters and melt into a supported child's pose or legs on a cushion pose. I have examples of both poses on my YouTube channel.

Pain management stretching breaks

The above-mentioned yoga routine is one example of a great way to use targeted yoga poses for pain relief. The more you play with different poses, the more tools you have in your arsenal for pain relief. I personally use neck stretches, cat and cow pose, supported child's pose, adjusted seated pigeon pose and adjusted dancer's pose for pain relief throughout the day.

With sleep, this is where the work on the nervous system, restorative yoga, and meditation shine. They can help with sleep from multiple angles. By taking appropriate rest breaks during the day and being less overtired at bedtime, we can make it easier to fall asleep. Calming the nervous system with restorative yoga and/or meditation at bedtime can help us to fall asleep faster. By doing guided meditation when we wake in the middle of the night we simultaneously enable deep rest. Don't worry so much about not being asleep and it can make it easier to go back to sleep.

During flares my go to is Yoga Nidra guided meditation. If I can get pain relief, my heating pad and a Yoga Nidra meditation all together, I can usually function again pretty quickly. With four children, I need flares not to take me out fully. It is the most efficient way I have to manage flares. When pain and fatigue levels are high, I do Yoga Nidra twice a day where possible.

We can create a pretty full symptom management toolkit using yoga tools alone. Thankfully we have a heap more to add as well. The more tools the better. Five-minute rescues are a big part of my management plan when life is too full for proper treatment plans. On days where I could not rest due to the children, I would do five-minute meditations on the couch or in my room with the door open while they were occupied. I have done five-minute stretching breaks with the baby climbing on my back as I do it.

I hope you have got a sense from this chapter of all the ways yoga could potentially help you.

Resource List

My YouTube channel has several classes including bed yoga, seated yoga, and meditation classes.

I offer a free series called Yoga for Chronic Pain and Fatigue which gives you an overview of the four key tools I love and use.

The Foundations of Yoga for Chronic Pain and Fatigue is a full program designed to help you learn or adapt your yoga practice with chronic pain and fatigue. You can find more information through my website.

Action Points

Sign up for my free Yoga for Chronic Pain and Fatigue series to try all four key tools. You can also find it at:

BOOK GOODIE BAG

How I Use Gentle Exercise As A Tool

One rule of fighting Fibromyalgia is to keep moving, even when it seems near impossible. If stretching is all you can manage, do it. If you can walk down your hallway and back, do it. If you can do a series of Yoga Sun Salutations, do it.

Movement keeps the muscles moving and strong. It's much harder to bring the muscles back from atrophy than it is to keep using them.

Of course, I don't mean you should be launching into graded exercise therapy and pushing your way up to functional improvements to the detriment of your quality of life. Quality of life is what all of this is about.

I once saw a physiotherapist who was very pleased with himself because a patient with chronic back pain doubled the amount he was able to walk each day, without decreasing his pain levels. I wondered what the patient considered success. Personally, walking more than the minimum heart health recommendations every day without symptom improvement wouldn't be "success".

A meta-analysis of the impact of aerobic exercise on Fibromyalgia symptoms revealed positive impacts on pain, fatigue, and mood. However, the effects were lost post treatment. Exercise must be done regularly to continue to see the benefit (see Winfried Häuser et al's article *Efficacy of Different Types of Aerobic Exercise in Fibromyalgia Syndrome*).

It is recommended that we begin below our ability level and then build up slowly. The goal of exercise is to improve our quality of life. Therefore, increasing your exercise capacity but leaving pain levels similar or increased, is not considered success. The quote below from the article *Exercise Therapy for Fibromyalgia* (2011) explains the best method:

"The intensity and duration of exercise sessions should be reduced when significant post-exertion pain or fatigue is experienced, and the intensity increased by 10% after 2 weeks of exercise without exacerbating symptoms."

Moderate intensity exercise is usually recommended. Warm water exercise is particularly helpful due to the water providing a weightlessness. Walking, strength training and yoga are all regularly recommended types of exercise. The most important choice here is a type of exercise that you like and will do.

A part of learning to use exercise more effectively in my fibromyalgia journey was reducing the amount I did. I pushed myself for years because I enjoy it and I was accidentally creating more pain. When I reduced my exercise to short walks, I decreased the pain in my gluteus area and legs significantly. Over a period of a couple of years I found that my sweet spot was a daily 20-minute walk. This was enjoyable at the time and did not trigger post-exertion pain or fatigue. Once a week I did a longer walk. I also learnt to reduce the tension from my exercise. My physiotherapist at the time, who was also a Pilates instructor, taught me to keep my neck down during classes in order to release the strain on my highly activated neck muscles. Just because we can do something, doesn't mean we should. It is good to seek expert advice. Likewise, a few years later, when I sought help from a yoga teacher to create a personalised routine, much of the personalisation involved amending poses to be less strenuous on my body.

When we use movement properly it becomes another tool for our toolkit. If one area is particularly tight, stretches may help. If we are tight, wound up, and overwhelmed a gentle walk may serve. Our choice of movement, wisely carried out, can soothe our mood, the nervous system, reduce pain, boost energy, and more.

We will talk more in the next chapter about how to approach exercise with chronic pain and fatigue.

How To Start Exercising With Chronic Pain And Fatigue

We are often told to start exercising when we have chronic pain and fatigue. But we aren't really told how to do it safely and without increasing our symptoms. This often results in patients doing too much with no help or guidance and they end up exacerbating their symptoms or hurt so much, they become wary of doing any exercise.

The amount of exercise you do depend on what your goals are for your exercise as well as what you can do safely without making yourself worse. I love yoga because it's got some great side benefits. I am all about improving my quality of life. I would rather exercise for 10 good minutes and see symptom improvement, than the "recommended" amounts and see no improvement – or worse, an increase in symptoms.

Assuming you are cleared for movement by your medical team, and you have discussed what you should avoid, the first recommendation is to start low and go slow. Take where you think you are able to start and reduce that by about 30%. Be mindful and listen to your body. Approach it like an experiment.

Does it feel good at the time? How do you feel after your practice? And how do you feel over the next couple of days?

Track your symptoms and exercise as you go.

When I was resuming exercise after significant pelvis and mobility issues during my third pregnancy, I began with walking around my backyard. Next, I tried walking to the end of my street and back. Each time, I assessed how I felt. When I was ready, I added a little more to the walk. Over a period of a few months, I built up to 40-minute walks with a break in the middle at the park with the children. It is important to note that this was not a linear progression. Some days, either my pain or fatigue levels meant that I reduced the amount I did. On others, I'd realise in the middle of the walk that it was too far and I would have increased pain for a couple of days. This isn't science! There are many factors involved.

As I suggested in the previous chapter, do what you will like and do. If we don't like it, why would we prioritise it when we are tired and in pain all the time? Take some time to find what you like and then commit to it to make it a habit.

Remember that it is quality not quantity. You are better off doing one great push-up than 10 poor-quality ones. The concept works with yoga, walking, and anything else. Do less with good form so you don't add to your bodily stress and tension.

Yoga for Fibromyalgia Framework

My framework for yoga for fibromyalgia is to breathe, stretch, and rest. I believe in working with the central nervous system, not against it. In this way our exercise becomes a multi-use tool.

Also, I would argue the breathing and resting are more important than the stretching portion. But the beauty of this framework is that you can adapt it to your energy levels and needs on any given day.

5 minutes to breathe, 5 minutes to stretch, 10 minutes to rest

2 minutes to breathe, 6 minutes to stretch, 2 minutes to rest

Those minutes of stretching can also be done on a bed, chair, or the mat. I am known for doing standing poses while the children are playing on the playground. It is about fitting it into our lives and doing what works.

My Physical Therapy Of Choice: Physiotherapy And Acupuncture

You can learn to do a lot for yourself, but a good treatment with a compassionate, knowledgeable practitioner is truly a blessing. My physiotherapist is the only person I tell most of my daily symptoms to. It's a gift to speak it out loud and have someone understand.

Research appears to be mixed about the benefits of acupuncture on Fibromyalgia symptoms. An analysis undertaken in 2013 *(Acupuncture for Treating Fibromyalgia* on PubMed)* looked at nine trials with 395 participants and found this:

"Acupuncture is probably better than non-acupuncture treatment in reducing pain and stiffness and improving overall well-being and fatigue; acupuncture without electrical stimulation probably does not reduce pain or improve fatigue, overall well-being or sleep."

Traditional acupuncture didn't help me either, but the use of acupuncture needles in trigger points does. In the case of trigger points, a lot of support appears for treatment by a physical therapist. In the article Information About Trigger Points and Their Treatment (n.d.), it states:

"Doctors may use local anaesthetic, saline, or cortisone injections, but acupuncture needling, use of a cold spray whilst stretching the muscle, or specific trigger point massage also works. Some physiotherapists or masseurs have a real knack in treating TPs [trigger point]."

Recently, I learnt after over a decade that my neck pain is caused by MPS: severe, recurring trigger points. Acupuncture needles in the trigger points in my neck and shoulders help me to the point that I cannot go too long without treatment. Nothing else will hold off the increasing pain and tension, which results in dizziness, nausea, and severe headaches.

Find a physical therapy that offers you, with your unique experience. relief. Some key physical therapies are physiotherapy, massage, osteopathy, chiropractic, and reflexology.

Through a lot of experience, research, trial and error, I know that I need neck tractions and stretches before and after acupuncture needles are placed into the trigger points on my sub occipital and upper trapezius points.

I use self-trigger point therapy by using a peanut ball or Theracane trigger point massager, and I stretch regularly. I also do all of the things I write about in this book. I ply my neck with heat in the form of hot showers, heat packs, and non-medicated hot rubs.

Still, I need to see the physiotherapist for this treatment within three weeks or I begin to struggle with sleep. The pain and tightness will keep me awake, drive me to change pillows multiple times, turn on the heating pad repeatedly, and, if necessary, take medicine.

I always start the day stiff, but when my neck is worse, it can be so stiff and tight that I can hardly move it, and the accompanying headache is relentless. If I let it escalate too far, then I'll end up miserable and unable to function. At this level, only muscle relaxants work.

I am thankful I have worked this out. It enables me to limit the pain relief medications I need to take as well as improve my quality of life. Try to take some time to find what may provide you with relief. Some people swear by regular massages, others by osteopathy. I have found that a lot of these therapies overlap. My physiotherapist can do some chiropractic adjustments if needed and an osteopath will utilise massage, craniosacral therapy, and adjustments, too.

I love physiotherapy for fibromyalgia. My physiotherapist is great. She is very qualified and also committed to learning about fibromyalgia, which is rare for any type of professional.

She does a type of gentle dry needling where she inserts acupuncture needles into trigger points in my neck and lets them sit there to encourage blood flow for around 15 minutes. While the needles are in, she uses ultrasound on muscles in my lower back and glutes.

The effect is gently released trigger points and muscles. It is the only treatment that has ever made a long-term difference, and I've tried many types of treatments.

How many times have you gone to a new physical

treatment provider and had trouble explaining what you need? Or you explain it but they don't really know what to do? Or, worse, they jump in, guns blazing, and cause a severe flare for the next week?

Too many to count for me. And when you just need some help, and the help turns to hurt, it's hard to manage.

Here are the two things that my physiotherapist understands that I wish all physical therapists understood:

First, I wish they understood the complex interplay of trigger points, chronic pain, chronic fatigue and the central nervous system. All patients are different.

Chronic pain on its own is a different ballgame to chronic pain with chronic fatigue. A sensitive central nervous system impacts everything, down to how you react to stimuli. The interplay of our symptoms is complex and unique. This must be understood and is something I consider in every yoga class I create.

Treatment for trigger points will vary when one has a central nervous system sensitivity. I have been to a physiotherapist who jabbed at the trigger points making them jump violently. They may have released, temporarily, but the jolt to my nervous system jammed everything back up. I was in a flare for over a week.

Second, I wish they understood how their treatment might cause a flare.

Following on from the above-mentioned points their treatments can cause suffering if they are not careful. In order to consider their treatment plan, they need to understand all of the above.

For example, I had to wait three months between treatments during lockdown, so on the first appointment back my physiotherapist may have wanted to go hard to release all of the tension causing me debilitating pain and headaches. But she knew going hard would make everything worse. So, she moderated her treatment to this knowledge and made life more tolerable for me.

As a bonus, and a way to get the most from my appointments, she always leaves me with suggestions for home management.

So next time you're considering a new physical therapist, maybe sound out their understanding of these two points.

Finding Relief From Pain

This chapter has been more than 20 years in the making. This book is a love song to all the things I do that help. This chapter will focus on all the ways I know to ease pain. This journey will be one I continue for the rest of my life.

The great news is that many of the tools I use hit multiple symptoms. For example, Yoga Nidra helps me with sleep, fatigue, pain, headaches (even severe ones) and more. It has helped calm my central nervous system overactivation over a period of several years which is key to calming the whole of our symptoms. I share more about this You can't control pain well without first reducing what causes or amplifies the pain. There is no point popping pills if you are not taking care of yourself. Most of the things I do to be well are basic healthy living guidelines.

I have lived with constant pain for a long time. I don't remember a time without pain. The only time I have minimal pain messages is right after a Yoga Nidra meditation. It's that part in meditation where you are neither awake nor asleep, but your physical body is profoundly relaxed. That is my favourite part of my day. Pain interferes with daily activities and sleep. Managing pain permeates every aspect of my life. But I have managed to halve my average pain levels and I live with a lot less pain daily than I did before this journey began. This requires a multi-pronged approach in terms of the big things that include proper sleep, medicines that help, pacing, good rest, and more. Then there are the band aid fixes, and the reactions to pain as it occurs. The lists below start with the big things and then move onto these smaller, everyday things.

A pain management plan is a good place to start. Write down all the things that help you already and continue to do them regularly. Then create a list of things you'd like to try. Slowly work your way through this list. A flare management plan is also a useful document to create. Write down the things that help you when symptoms are skyrocketing. These are the things you need to do when it's getting too hard to manage your usual daily activities.

My Specific Regimen

Focusing on lifestyle, I'll start with sleep. Sleep affects pain levels like nobody's business. I have a comprehensive sleep hygiene plan that I follow, and this includes medicine. For more information, see the chapter The Foundation Upon Which All Is Built: Sleep.

Keep moving even when it seems near impossible. Refer to the chapter How I Use Gentle Exercise As A Tool.

Incorporating rest into the day is necessary. Regular periods of rest with my heat pack reduce the amount of pain at bedtime, making it easier to get to sleep. A 20–30-minute meditation is more refreshing than attempting to nap and it is one of the best tools I have in my arsenal.

Pacing is using the energy and pain levels we have wisely. I work part-time. Work-life balance must include your personal context. Note that managing children or other caregiving needs also count as work hours.

Reduce or remove perpetuating factors. Identify the things that exacerbate your symptoms and try to reduce or remove them.

Try to see food as fuel and, therefore, nourish yourself appropriately.

Specific Options For Pain Relief

Low dose Naltrexone. It is part of my whole lifestyle plan for wellness. It has changed everything for me.

For a long time, the only thing I had was a low dose of amitriptyline. It would help me get to sleep where nothing else worked. It also helped with some of the widespread pain.

Recovery Factors amino acid supplement

My heat pack is my first line of defence. I use it on my neck first thing, whenever I can during the day, in the evening and at bedtime.

If I can't use my heat pack or I cannot sit around with it, I will use Deep Heat, a non-medicated heat-producing rub that eases muscle pain, especially when combined with a good massage.

A hot bath is my best treat and the first thing I want when the pain increases.

MSM (Methylsulfonylmethane) for muscle and joint pain. It helped with the pain in my index fingers during the coldest months as well as my neck.

Ibuprofen or paracetamol (Acetaminophen) for headaches or low-level pain

A muscle relaxant for spasms in the neck or back. The frequency of these has decreased since I began LDN.

I see the physiotherapist every two or three weeks and they do neck tractions/mobilisations and place acupuncture needles in trigger points in my neck and shoulders. This is the only thing that keeps my neck free and helps the severe headaches, dizziness, and nausea that accompany severe neck pain.

A Theracane trigger point massager and peanut ball for self-trigger point release

Magnesium oil

Some Natural Pain Relief Methods

- Heat pack
- Ice pack
- Hot bath or shower
- For a bad headache, put your feet in hot water and an ice pack around your neck
- For headaches or muscle tension, use Peppermint oil on the temples mixed with a carrier oil such as coconut oil, which is less greasy than other oils. Lavender oil massaged into your feet or neck/temples if you can handle the smell

- Check all nutrient levels and supplements where needed – especially magnesium and iron
- Meditation
- Yoga routines for chronic illness
- Cat and cow pose
- Self-trigger-point work
- Acupressure release
- Theracane trigger point massager
- Peanut ball
- Foam roller
- Rest and sleep – get as much as possible
- Physiotherapy with acupuncture – especially for trigger points
- Massage: self-massage, partner/friend massage or paid massage
- Herbal topical relief cream such as arnica-based creams or Deep Heat
- Gentle walks might seem counterproductive but often helps my neck and back. The key word is gentle.
- Distraction with funny videos or calling a friend
- Stretching. I cannot stress this enough. Stretch several times a day.

Teas/Infusions with potential benefits:
- Turmeric
- Thyme
- Chamomile
- Nettle

- Red Raspberry Leaf

Supplements
- MSM
- Curcumin
- Recovery Factors
- Energy Revitalisation Formula
- FibroMalic (Malic acid)
- Magnesium
- Fish oil
- Acetyl L-carnitine
- 5-HTP (not to be taken with some medications such as antidepressants)
- SAMe (not to be taken with some medications such as antidepressants)

Action Points

Create a list of things that already help you with your pain. Make a list of things you would like to try and discuss with your doctor. I have included a printable list of fibromyalgia treatments in the book goodie bag. Create a daily Pain Management Plan and a Flare Plan for when symptoms escalate. The Ultimate Wellbeing Planner Kit, which includes both a Pain Management Plan and Flare Plans, which can also be purchased from www.melissavsfibromyalgia.com/book/

All I Had For A Long Time: Amitriptyline

As I mentioned, prior to LDN, amitriptyline was the only thing to help me sleep.

The mechanism of amitriptyline is to increase the level of serotonin, which is hypothesized to be low in people with Fibromyalgia.

In *Fibromyalgia and Muscle Pain: Your Guide to Self-Treatment* (2015) by Leon Chaitow ND, DO, the section on medication is very small, but he does mention amitriptyline as one of the most useful medicines prescribed for Fibromyalgia.

"Studies involving various forms of antidepressant medication tend to support the use of amitriptyline (25 to 50 mg daily), with pain scores, stiffness, sleep and fatigue symptoms all improving on average, but by no means in all sufferers."

I was put on amitriptyline before I was diagnosed by a locum GP I saw only once. Without knowing what it does or why I was put on it, it turned out to be the best foundation for my journey to wellness. I started on 50mg per night and stayed on this dose until I questioned its efficacy. One clue was I slept poorly, and my Fitbit sleep chart was always alight with the colours of restlessness or awake time. I barely cobbled together an hour of sleep at a time.

One December, I decided to experiment with going off it. I slowly reduced my dose because this is not a medicine that you can just stop. I went much more slowly than my doctor suggested, and this served me well. On the way down, I noted that at 30mg and 25mg, I experienced the same level of benefit with sleep at my 50mg dose. When I got lower than that, I began to sleep extremely poorly, to feel a lot more pain, and I got constant headaches. I endured two weeks completely off it, including trialling 5HTP, a supplement said to help with sleep, and I was miserable.

Declaring amitriptyline as useful, I went back to 25mg. It was a good thing to have tested its worth after nearly a decade on it because there are side effects and risks. However, learning I could halve the dose was a good lesson.

In 2018, after the birth of my third baby, I decided to stop taking it as I was confident the LDN was helping enough, and I was going to experience sleep deprivation anyway because of the baby. I quietly stopped taking it, unsure if it would stick. After a week, I acknowledged to myself that I was ok. I then announced it to my husband – I was so excited to finally be off a medicine I didn't feel I needed anymore after more than a decade on it. I am thankful it helped me when nothing else did but with LDN, the cost vs benefit analysis no longer worked for me.

When my doctor and I discuss treatments for migraines, Amitriptyline often comes up again. This is because it is a well-studied medicine that has extra side benefits for me with helping with sleep. I would rather try a medicine I have already been on with success, and tolerable side effects. However, I would also rather not take a long-term medicine if I don't need to. There is a new cost-benefit analysis needed for every situation.

The Trick With Supplements

Supplements are a tricky area to write about. Requirements are very individual. There are several supplements that are broadly recommended for Fibromyalgia patients. However, a lot of them are a waste of money, unless your body needs them.

Dr Teitelbaum, Dr Liptan, Dr Brady, and numerous other doctors writing books and articles about Fibromyalgia recommend liberal use of supplements and natural remedies. Anecdotally, patients will swear by certain ones.

Unless you have a good functional medicine doctor or naturopath who can do reliable testing and tell you exactly what your body needs, you're flying blind.

As a person who has tried a lot of supplements based upon research, doctors' recommendations and a disappointing naturopath who encouraged me to spend hundreds of dollars to be cured, I can tell you what I take. There are countless articles to wade through. Here, I outline some articles recommending supplements for Fibromyalgia.

Some of the most mentioned supplements are:

Acetyl L-carnitine	Turmeric and black pepper
Magnesium	Vitamin D3
Fish oil	5-HTP

SAMe

CoQ10 (energy)

D-Ribose (energy)

In his article *8 Natural Ways to Overcome Fibromyalgia Symptoms* (n.d.), Dr Axe lists the main symptoms of Fibromyalgia, treatment options, foods to eat to gain good nutrients, such as melatonin, and natural treatments. Karen Lee Richards discusses the diminished energy present for those with Fibromyalgia and lists several options in her article *8 Energy-Boosting Supplements for Fight Fibromyalgia Fatigue* (2011) on the Fibromyalgia Treatment Group website. On that same website, there's an article called 10 Herbs and Supplements to Try for Fibromyalgia Pain (n.d.), and it focuses on pain and adds Alpha Lipoic Acid, Rhodiola Rosea and Butterbur in addition to the list above.

Fibro Daze's article *14 Supplements That May Help Fibromyalgia* (2014) diverges a little from the other articles and adds malic acid, B complex, NADH, DHEA, probiotics, and melatonin. The author, Sue, who has Fibromyalgia, takes these alongside a multivitamin and milk thistle.

Dr Teitelbaum's website EndFatigue.com has a Nutrition Guide with a list of herbals, vitamins, minerals, and other supplements with links to further information about them and recommended dosage.

I have read Dr Teitelbaum's books and a lot of the articles on his website and it all makes sense to me. I feel I would have made more progress if doctors would help me tackle the sleep issue. He believes, if necessary, that a couple of low dose medicines to aid sleep for several months is very efficacious to healing[30]. As I've mentioned, I like his book From *Fatigued to Fantastic* (2021).

The two key supplements I take are:

- Magnesium
- Recovery Factors (amino acid supplement)

I also like:

- Moringa Powder for nutritional support. It has 18 amino acids and it's a good source of vitamins and minerals.
- MSM
- B-complex
- A multi-vitamin

It is a good idea when trying new supplements to add one thing at a time and to track the outcomes. Please keep in mind, it does take time for these to build up in the system.

[30] Dr. Jacob Teitelbaum. (2013). *The Fatigue and Fibromyalgia Solution*. Avery.

Amino Acid Supplementation

Amino acid supplementation and other medical foods for fibromyalgia appear to be a useful treatment option.

This article about nutritional management of fibromyalgia states that: *"Patients with sleep disorders demonstrate a nutritional deficiency of tryptophan, choline and GABA. Fibromyalgia patients also have reduced blood levels of serotonin and 5-hydroxytryptophan. A double-blind, randomized trial compared an amino acid based medical food with trazodone to study sleep latency and parasympathetic autonomic nervous system improvement in sleeping hours. The results showed improved sleep quality without morning grogginess along with improved night-time parasympathetic activity with the use of the medical food."*[31]

We know sleep is huge in fibromyalgia. It is a massive perpetuating factor. We also know that the nervous system is an important part of our puzzle.

Amino acids can help everything, *"From treating sleep disorders and energy deficits to nervous system and methylation factors that support proper neutralizing and elimination of toxins*

---

[31] Nutritional Management of Fibromyalgia
http://www.archivesofmedicine.com/medicine/nutritional-management-of-fibromyalgia.php?aid=9131

within the body."[32]

At the end of 2019 Doctor Teitelbaum offered an opportunity to try a supplement that he and a fellow doctor had been finding helpful with their fibromyalgia patients. Recovery Factors is a porcine serum polypeptide extract that is used in hospitals for patients with severe malnutrition.

As one of the lucky participants I received my bottles and started the trial eagerly.

I noticed that the ingredients label listed iron and an extensive list of amino acids. Iron is something I have been deficient in my entire adult life, even when I ate more meat.

The first few nights I took the full dose as recommended and slept like I was heavily sedated. When I woke up my neck was very sore from immobility, and I had a severe headache.

After struggling through a few days feeling more and more lethargic, I emailed Doctor Teitelbaum's office asking if I should decrease the dose. Doctor T himself replied that I should and take the dose that works for me.

I reduced it to half and continued to sleep better but less heavily. I noticed less gut issues, slightly less pain, and slightly more energy.

The bottles lasted me longer due to my dosage. I wanted to prolong it even more, so I dropped down to two pills at bedtime only. I continued to sleep better.

In March 2020 I ran out of them and then the lockdown happened in New Zealand. I ended up with no supplement, no

[32] Treatments for Fibromyalgia: Amino Acid Therapy https://www.living-smarter-with-fibromyalgia.com/treatment-for-fibromyalgia-amino-acids.html

physiotherapy, a lot of stress, no childcare and a new job. My sleep deteriorated. The migraines, of which I'd had two the previous month and one a year prior, escalated.

In June my doctor and I agreed I'd go back on Amitriptyline for a time, and I'd order the Recovery Factors supplement which was now for sale.

In addition, for the first time in many years I have nearly optimal iron levels without iron injections. This is important for me as I tend to live at the very bottom of a very big range and I feel the effects. I get lethargic, fatigued and dizzy.

Recovery Factors helps me with sleep. Sleep leads to less pain and fatigue. This, in turn, leads to better enjoyment of life, more ability to do what I want to do (higher functionality), and better sleep. It's like a reversal of the vicious cycle of fibromyalgia. I am not healed, but I am doing more of what I want with less pain and fatigue.

The results are out from the Porcine Serum Polypeptide Nutritional Supplement study[33] and they found :

- 69.5% average increase in energy
- 69.2% average increase in overall well being
- 54.1% average improvement in sleep
- 60.5% average improvement in mental clarity
- 37.9% average decrease in discomfort
- 34.8% average improvement in calmness
- 54.6% average improvement in digestive symptoms

These are very promising results and align with my

[33] Nutritional Intervention in Chronic Fatigue Syndrome and Fibromyalgia (CFS/FMS) A Unique Porcine Serum Polypeptide Nutritional Supplement
https://openpainjournal.com/VOLUME/13/PAGE/52/FULLTEXT/

experience. Though it is worth noting that the outcomes were self-reported therefore very subjective.

It is not cheap to have Recovery Factors shipped to New Zealand. But the cost, at my dosage, works out to be equivalent to a bottle of a good quality multivitamin each month, and gives me far better results. This has remained a key part of my protocol.

Headaches, Migraines, And Fibromyalgia

Headaches seem to go hand in hand with fibromyalgia. I experienced severe, debilitating headaches for a decade before a doctor finally realised they were migraines.

I was a routine appointment when I explained that I had had another headache so bad that I felt sick. I had to have my in-laws come and take the children so I could go to bed.

On the occasions that I wake with headaches this bad, I can only manage Panadol Soluble (acetaminophen/paracetamol) and then go back to my dark room with my heating pad, eye mask, and a Yoga Nidra meditation playing quietly.

Sometimes I don't realise I am in so much pain until I am vomiting in the toilet with small children watching. When they are this bad, I cannot function through them. This is difficult with small children. After a morning of sleeping through it, I can usually re-join the world but only if the curtains are drawn and everything is quiet. I tend to spend most of the time prodrome and postdrome (pre- and post-migraine) saying, "shhh" to my children. Postdrome periods feel like I'm hungover, leaving my exhausted, dehydrated, and generally wiped out.

Here is where it gets confusing! On other days I can develop a headache that feels bad enough for me to want to go to bed, but I can continue to function. Sometimes over the counter medicines are enough to continue my day. Sometimes they are not. It's a mixed bag. I thought that these were just bad headaches as opposed to migraine.

It turns out loads of people with fibromyalgia also experience migraine. In the study *Fibromyalgia and Headache: An epidemiological study supporting migraine as part of the fibromyalgia syndrome*, they found 76% of patients with fibromyalgia experienced chronic headaches. Migraine was diagnosed in 63% of fibromyalgia patients. They suggest that *"General measures of pain, pain-related disability, sleep quality, and psychological distress were similar in fibromyalgia patients with and without headache. Therefore, fibromyalgia patients with headache do not appear to represent a significantly different subgroup compared to fibromyalgia patients without headache."*[34]

There are differing types of headaches with different perpetuating factors. It can be difficult to determine what causes headaches and what is caused by them. For example, headaches can be caused by active trigger points in the neck and upper back. Sometimes these headaches cause the types of symptoms that occur with migraine, such as nausea, dizziness, and sensitivity to light and noise. The tricky part here is that migraines can also cause stiffness and pain in the neck.

I have experienced headaches to varying degrees over the years. Sometimes the only symptom is head pain. However, I find headaches harder to function through the other types of

---

[34] Fibromyalgia and Headache: an epidemiological study supporting migraine as part of the fibromyalgia syndrome

pain. So, they have been quite disruptive for me.

Some common symptoms that go along with severe headaches included:[35]

- Pain in various areas of the head and shoulders
- Nausea and/or vomiting
- Loss of balance
- Sensitivity to stimuli such as light, sound and smells
- If it is migraine then the following symptoms may also occur:
- Severe fatigue
- Brain fog
- Inability to sleep
- Joint stiffness
- Hangover affect post-headache

You can likely see why it is difficult to ascertain where fibromyalgia symptoms end, and headaches begin.

My doctor recommended I begin tracking my symptoms more carefully to try and assess triggers for migraine and to manage my day-to-day pain better. It was difficult for me to decide when pain was going to escalate into migraine or if it would ebb again. This took some real work.

There are quite a few treatments for migraine. Some crossovers with fibromyalgia and others do not. There are some great articles online about migraine medicines.

After trying to manage the migraine with over-the-counter medicines, we moved onto a triptan, which is an anti-nausea

---

[35] Fibromyalgia Chronic Headaches Causes, Symptoms, Treatments

medicine. I had been dealing with such severe headache and pain levels for so long it was difficult for me to know early enough in the attack to take the medicine.

Amitriptyline, a tricyclic antidepressant discussed earlier, is useful for fibromyalgia pain and the sedating effects can help with insomnia. It can also prevent migraine. Given the potential to help both conditions, my doctor suggested we try it again. I was hesitant as the side effects are a heavy consequence with this medicine. However, there are side effects associated with every medication available.

I tried the supplement combination recommended for migraine for a time – COQ10, B2 and Magnesium – to little noted effect. I was trying to manage the perpetuating factors as best I could, such as sleep, rest, neck and shoulder trigger points, etc.

This is just the beginning of this part of my journey. I am learning continually. What was surprising was that even though I had already been struggling with these for years without an extra diagnosis, I still felt a profound sense of grief for the new word. For the extra research and information gathering I needed to do and the new triggers and treatments I had to figure out.

The moral of the story is to keep tracking your symptoms and keep bringing things up with your medical team. Don't let things be shoved into the fibromyalgia basket because it causes unnecessary extra suffering.

The Brain (Fibro) Fog

There's a pernicious symptom of living with Fibromyalgia that can fall into the background of the twin peaks of pain and fatigue. It's something that affects our everyday lives, and we may not even realise it is a thing.

Brain fog or cognitive dysfunction can strike during any conversation, any task, and at any time.

I can't do confrontations because the stress causes me to forget how to stand up for myself. All the words or well-articulated statements I'd have written down become buried in fog when I try to access them in the moment. Even subjects I'm well researched on become minefields when reaching through my memory for the information. This is one reason I write everything down.

There's been a thousand conversations where I'm reaching for simple words that blew away a moment before I wanted them. There have been even more times when I say one thing when I mean another. Sometimes I know I've done it, but often I don't. Occasionally, I'll realise later. As someone who loves words and writing, it's more than a little upsetting.

Brain fog was thought to be another thing that is all in our heads, but *"a 2015 study in Arthritis Care and Research found that fibro fog is a real issue. In a study of 60 individuals – 30 with fibromyalgia and 30 without fibromyalgia – researchers found various impairments of attention and memory in fibromyalgia patients when compared with healthy controls. What remains unclear is what is causing the cognitive challenges"* (*Fibro Fog: Sleep, Brain Dysfunction Likely Culprits for Cognitive Difficulties Associated with Fibromyalgia*, the Arthritis Foundation website). It is thought as many as 50% of Fibromyalgia patients struggle with it, perhaps more.

Brain fog has been theorized to be caused by poor sleep, the nervous system being off-kilter, stress and anxiety, and pain severity. Though, they really don't know the cause yet.

Here's the ways it can manifest:

- Clumsiness/loss of spatial awareness
- Losing words
- Mixing up words
- Forgetting things
- Confusion Feeling overwhelmed Becoming easily distracted

Here's some things that help minimise brain fog:

- Get the best sleep you can
- Pace activity and rest
- Manage pain
- Give yourself time and understanding

These are not small things for us to do. I spend a lot of time working on good sleep and managing pain, and brain fog is still a big factor in my life. However, it's far better than what it was when I was at my worst.

Here's some ways to combat brain fog's effects:

Write it all down! Even before I was diagnosed or had any idea of why life was so much harder for me, I planned religiously and had lists upon lists.

Routines, automatic pilot can be useful

Explain it to those around you often

Check your medicines are not the culprits, sometimes our medicines cause as many issues as they solve; it's good to be aware of what their side effects are so we can mitigate them.

Brain fog is just one of those things that come with chronic sleep deprivation, pain, and fatigue, but there are many things we can do to compensate for it.

The Fibromyalgia and
Food Conundrum

A lot of Fibromyalgia fighters swear by eating one way or the other. I have found that prioritising whole foods has been the only answer for me. I tried gluten free for eight weeks to no effect. I am currently mostly dairy free as it upsets my tummy.

I have investigated vegetarianism, paleo, anti-inflammatory, and the other diets recommended for Fibromyalgia and have noticed one main similarity: prioritising vegetables is of the utmost importance even if they are low carb ones.

In her book *The Whole Health Life* (2016), Shannon Harvey writes about being well while living with a chronic illness that affects her gut. In her chapter on food, she outlines her research into the different diets and concludes that I agree with: "*A diet rich in whole, plant-based foods is the way to go.*"

I believe it is worth doing a trial excluding certain foods, especially gluten, as I have heard enough stories of partial or full recovery for it to be worth an eight-week trial. The Mediterranean Diet is highly regarded because it prioritises fresh fruits and vegetables, whole grains, healthy fats, seafood, and meats. You might like to research that further. For myself, my constant refrain is "food as fuel", thus I need the energy for living and don't want to waste valuable calories or risk allergies from trying to process junk food. I focus on vegetables, fruits, whole grains, protein, etc., but I am not super strict. I have found no foods that make me feel noticeably better by avoiding them. Aside from MSG, aspartame, and other chemicals/fake foods, I don't eliminate foods unless they cause an intolerance or allergy for me or are of no nutritional value.

Several years ago, I realised that my body was trying to gain energy by driving me to consume a lot of carbohydrates. Ironically, carbohydrates take lots of energy to process, thereby draining us of more energy and making me crave more food. By taking note of the food, I was eating on a daily basis for a few weeks, I realised that I was consuming way too many carbohydrates, especially the white ones with little to no nutritional value. The food diary showed me I was perpetuating a boom-bust cycle every few hours. I'd eat carbohydrates, crash, consume again, and crash again. When the fatigue increases, I notice a craving for the white carbs, especially Chelsea buns. It's been so obviously beneficial to me to avoid these, that it's usually not my first craving. But if it is, I easily make a swap for something better.

Sugar is another thing we consume too abundantly, especially. when we are tired. As opposed to trying to put myself on a strict diet to avoid sugar, I choose to focus on better food choices. By prioritising those foods mentioned above such as vegetables, fruits and whole grains, we leave less room for those processed, sugary, empty calorie, anti-nutrients we call food. As someone with a lot of coping mechanisms to enact every day, it is better to not make food a battleground.

It is worthwhile to experiment with this. I don't think food will be a cure, but it is helping us to get out of our own way by improving our fuel and digestion. If you are considering a more restrictive diet then do seek support from a qualified person to help you ensure you are meeting your nutritional needs.

Support Worksheet

Who can I talk to?

What's my plan for harder days?

Where can I go for support/information?

What I Do:
Morning Stiffness

Morning stiffness is a characteristic symptom of Fibromyalgia, arthritis, and rheumatism. An article on *Fibromyalgia Symptoms* website, morning stiffness and Fibromyalgia (n.d.), suggests that up to 90% of those with Fibromyalgia suffer from morning stiffness.

Morning stiffness means exactly what it sounds like. You wake up with stiff, aching muscles, usually in the neck and spine. It can last an hour or linger for the day.

My neck and spine usually stiffen up over the course of the night. Movement returns slowly over the morning. I am incapable of doing much exercise before lunchtime as my back will not cooperate and it's usually as stiff as a board.

The National Fibromyalgia and Chronic Pain Association website has an article *10 Tips to Relieve Morning Stiffness* (n.d.) by Roger Chu, PhD, LAc, QME, and this list includes some basic ideas such as exercise, getting enough sleep, avoiding getting too cold, eating healthier food, and having a plan for coping with stress.

I dislike references that assume weight, food, and exercise are the three big ways to address everything in Fibromyalgia. – I have eaten healthily, kept to a healthy weight range and exercised beyond the minimum requirements since long before I was diagnosed, and my symptoms didn't get much better. These are great whole of life tips, but they aren't going to magically cure things like morning stiffness or Fibromyalgia for that matter!

Five Ways I Cope With Morning Stiffness

Low Dose Naltrexone (LDN)

Prior to LDN, my neck would get progressively stiffer as the night continued, resulting in multiple pillow changes, medication, non-medicated warming rub, or my heat pack. By 5am, my neck would be too stiff to stay lying down, but my body was too exhausted to get up. Now, I can get through the night on one pillow, rarely take medication, and sometimes don't need to use a non-medicated warming rub such as Deep Heat.

Heat

Using my heat pack in the evening and applying it first thing in the morning are key for managing my neck. I also sleep with an electric heating pad that I turn on a few times per night, as needed. My neck requires almost 24/7 management. Heat is king. I set my children up with toast first thing so that I can sit with my heat pack and coffee. If I don't sit long enough my neck will remain stiff, tight, and sore all day. If you have time, a warm shower helps a lot!

Stretching

Stretching, specifically yoga poses, help get my spine moving. Seated cat/cow pose, chair sun salutations, half sun salutations or full sun salutations really help get my body moving. These are easily found in a Google search.

Deep Heat/Heated Rub

When I can no longer sit still with my heat pack, I'll use a heated rub. It has a strong smell, so it's not ideal, but it does help.

Slowly Get Going

I rarely take medicine prior to 10am as I find once the fatigue and first stiffness ease, I tend to feel better. So, I'll give my body some time to adjust to the day. If I had the time, a gentle walk would be ideal. My neck can occasionally be released by ibuprofen, spasms can be aided by a muscle relaxant, and headaches can sometimes be eased by paracetamol.

Morning stiffness is a common symptom, but there are plenty of things we can do to combat it.

How Do I Get Out Of Bed In The Morning With Chronic Pain/Fibromyalgia?

How can one make getting up with chronic pain and fatigue easier? It is difficult and many times over the last few years I've been thankful that I have to get up for my children. It's hard to get going when you don't wake feeling well.

I'd suggest using an alarm like a gently vibrating Fitbit. Give yourself some time to ease into the day. When you wake up, take some time to breathe gently. Once you're ready, ease yourself up, sit on the edge of your bed for a few moments and do some very gentle micro stretches. Whatever muscle is calling your attention loudest should get the most attention.

Making A Mindful Morning Routine

It might surprise you to know that I don't recommend diving into a yoga routine first thing in the morning. Our bodies are stiff and sore in the morning. However, some gentle stretches, breathing, and meditation can be a useful way to get going first thing in the morning

If you don't have to jump out of bed and directly into

151

managing multiple children, like me, then I suggest a mindful morning routine.

It could consist of a few moments of mindfulness when you first wake. Take some time to notice the light streaming in, the sounds you can hear, and the feel of the blanket on your body.

Stretch slowly, mindfully, and gently while still in bed.

You can try:

- Yoga Nidra guided meditation (Yes, right there in bed!)
- A breathing practice
- Gentle bed yoga
- Mindfulness meditation
- Seated stretches on the side of your bed
- Apply topical lotions while sitting on the side of your bed
- Use your peanut ball or other self-trigger point work Lie with your electric heating pad on while doing breathing or meditation for bonus points!

The sky's the limit. This is your morning, and you get to choose what works for you.

My Morning Routine

Like many of us, I have to just get up and go. I get the children organised and sit with my heat pack, toast and coffee. When I am getting dressed I do a few standing stretches.

I take mindful breathing breaks regularly. They are ingrained into my lifestyle. But I would absolutely incorporate some more time in bed for stretching and breathing if I could. Remember to ask what we can do.

The Best Way A Partner Can Support A Chronically Ill Person

Living with a chronic illness that causes unrelenting pain, fatigue, insomnia, and more is hard enough. It should be a given that if one has coping mechanisms that can reduce or limit the severity of these symptoms, they can do them. A partner should not be a barrier to symptom reducing coping mechanisms.

I have been living with these symptoms for more than 15 years. In the past several years I have managed to cut my pain and fatigue levels in half. But to do this I have to maintain some tight coping mechanisms.

These include not staying out late at night because symptoms get worse the more tired I get. By 10pm I am unequivocally finished with the day. The later I go to bed, the harder it is for me to sleep. This is a paradox that makes sleep restriction therapy hilariously sad. Getting less sleep means more pain and fatigue the next day.

It also includes ensuring I get time to do Yoga Nidra guided meditation in the day and other daily coping mechanisms such as stretching and heat application.

Pacing is a vital part of managing fibromyalgia symptoms

well. Pacing means alternating activity and rest in a manner congruent with pain and fatigue levels. This means knowing how much I am capable of without flaring my symptoms.

It is hard enough learning these lessons and to put them in place. It is also hard to miss out and create boundaries to manage my symptoms. I get frustrated and sad about what I would like to do.

But I also get frustrated and sad when coping with higher pain and fatigue levels when pushed past these boundaries.

What a partner needs to do is help me to keep these boundaries.

The best thing a partner can do when someone with fibromyalgia expresses the fact that something might be too much for them is to say, "How can we manage this so that you can experience it without feeling miserable at the time and afterward?"

The worst thing a partner can do is to invalidate your feelings, dismiss you, or regard you with derision when you say something will be difficult or too much.

The bottom line is a partner should want the best for their loved one. They should want their loved one to experience less pain and fatigue, while living a fulfilling life. It can be difficult for a partner to see when things are better or worse and it might appear that one can't influence it. This is where communication helps. Find a way to share when things are better or worse and recognize together that certain things help or hinder progress. I have found a straightforward conversation about the things I need that my husband can influence is a great start. We are in a phase of our lives that is heavily influenced by small children and their needs. The parameters in which to move are small, however there is always time for my husband to help me create space for a rest.

I am no expert; I am still trying to navigate my way through nurturing a marriage alongside small children and a chronic illness. One thing I am trying to get better at is speaking up for what I need and want, because I believe this ultimately helps our marriage.

This will look different for every relationship. It will be vastly different when a partner is also a caregiver. The fact remains that the best question a partner can ask on any given day, but particularly hard days is, "How can we manage this so that you can experience it without feeling miserable at the time and afterward?"

The Side Effect Of Chronic Illness No One Talks About

There's a side effect of living with chronic illness no one adds to the list of symptoms but is so pervasive it might even top pain. It's called trauma.

It is traumatic to live with conditions that cause such intense symptoms and such disruption. Not knowing how we will feel when we get up each day is traumatic. The loss of my late teen years and twenties to illness is still a source of grief.

This does not include the trauma of being gaslighted, ignored, and accused of making it up. It also doesn't include asking medical professionals for help and receiving inadequate care.

I've come a long way and I still get flashes of how bad it was. Times I felt completely helpless and alone. I remember how it was to be treated by doctors and specialists who couldn't or wouldn't help. I remember what it was like to feel so much pain and fatigue with no assistance. And when I flare, I internally panic it will go back to what it was. We never want those high symptoms to come back! This also does not account for the theory that trauma (big or small) can be a contributing factor to the development of Fibromyalgia. Things like illness, abuse, bullying, natural disasters, pregnancy, and more all induce trauma and trauma responses..

I strive to be positive, optimistic, thankful, prayerful, and focus on what I can do. It's good to acknowledge those feelings as they arise. Sit with them for a moment. They are a valid part of what makes us who we are.

Work with those feelings, speak with a counsellor, journal through them, meditate or pray on them. But don't ignore them.

Working With
Chronic Pain And Fatigue

How can I work with a chronic illness? How can I continue to work with a chronic illness? If you've ever asked yourself these questions, then this chapter is for you. Having run the gamut of ways to try to continue working with a chronic illness, I have learned a lot. In short, I do believe we can work with a chronic illness, but we need some support to do so.

Sometimes fibromyalgia, chronic pain and fatigue are defined as a disability. That depends on your location in the world. This article from Harvard Business Review states that:

"Over one-third of Europeans aged 15 years or older and nearly 60% of adult Americans are living with at least one chronic illness. Chronic illness can last from several months to a lifetime and can take many forms: arthritis, musculoskeletal pain, diabetes, asthma, migraine, blood disorders, cancer, heart disease, irritable bowel syndrome, autoimmune disease, and a range of mental illnesses like depression and debilitating anxiety. Each year, depression or anxiety account for up to 50% of chronic sick leave in Europe. Despite this omnipresence, leaders are overwhelmingly unprepared to support chronically ill

employees."[36]

It is high time to start supporting those who are chronically ill in their efforts to remain in the workforce or. Or there won't be a workforce.

Working From Home
For Chronic Illness Fighters

Energy conservation and the ability to administer self-care are two very important elements of living well with chronic illness. Working from home, while a little isolating, is a great opportunity for chronic illness fighters. When I was contracting, it was also a fantastic way to be flexible around my husband and baby.

When I first went part-time, I also reduced my commute from an hour each way on the bus to 30 minutes in my car. This can save a lot of energy on its own. When I was working after I had my first son, I still had to drive him to and from his carer's place, but at least I didn't have to fight my way into town afterwards.

It hasn't always been an option in my roles, but since the pandemic it's become a necessity to be able to work from home. And once you have proven that you can do your work well, it's worth building a case to continue.

One of the key reasons I love working from home is that I

[36] https://hbr.org/2021/02/how-managers-can-support-employees-with-chronic-illnesses

have the flexibility to do Yoga Nidra during my lunch breaks. This makes a big difference for pain and fatigue levels.

It is also easier to do your yoga and stretches when no one is watching. Set your timers and take your stretching breaks. Another thing you don't need to worry about hiding is your heat pack, smelly topical lotions and whatever else you use to manage pain during the workday. No one needs to know if you're wandering around during a meeting rather than sitting still.

You also have more control over your working area – temperature control, lighting, windows, etc. My home desk is set up perfectly for me and I have my Swiss ball if I get sick of my chair (this was basically the only way I could sit down for any length of time in the third trimester of all pregnancies – the back pain was unbelievable). With hot desking and inappropriately set up offices, it's a relief to have my ergonomically ideal monitor, stand, seat and footstool.

The cherry on the top for employers, and for yourself, is that you get more done without constant interruptions and without the little stressors the office provides. (Research suggests it takes something like half an hour to settle back into a task with each interruption.) This helps with productivity but also with brain fog.

These are the reasons I prefer to work from home (or a blend of office and homework) and could be good reasons for you to explore this as an option too.

In 2020, between the three kids and lockdowns, working from home made a massive difference for me. I was able to start my online yoga studio specifically for chronic pain and fatigue at the same time with little bits of work here and there. The three things that helped most were eliminating time to commute, having my workspace perfectly set up for my needs, and meditating in my lunch break.

Tips for Managing at Work

As a person who has worked in full time office jobs, worked part-time, worked from home, and created my own business, I can tell you that none is easy when you have a chronic illness. They are especially hard when your employer doesn't understand your condition and is not/cannot accommodate you.

The good news is that there are many things we can do ourselves to manage our work and our illness so I will share some ideas for you.

Ways to work with fibromyalgia, chronic pain, and fatigue

- Modifications to your workstation (ergonomic assessment)
- Use a discreet heating pad
- Have healthy snacks and loads of water
- Take appropriate breaks and implement micro breaks
- If you usually stand for work, try to sit during your

break and raise your legs if possible. If you usually sit, try to walk for part of your break.

- Use discreet regular stretches and full stretches where possible
- Meditation can be done during longer breaks and/right after work
- Breathe regularly
- Use your sick leave when you need it.
- Use the physical therapy that works for you

Flexible work options to negotiate:
- Reduced and/or flexible hours
- Set your hours to earlier or later according to your best energy envelope
- Working reduced hours Reducing one day a week
- A condensed work week may help some

Did you know that there are things you can do after work that can help you manage at work? Things like taking a break when you first get home from work can help immensely. I highly recommend Yoga Nidra, as you know, even for just 15 minutes. Stretch your key muscles and/or take a gentle walk if possible. Use your coping mechanisms and I also highly recommend your mindful bedtime routine to help relieve tension from the day, prepare for sleep and nourish the body ready for the next day.

How yoga can support you at work:

- Meditating in your breaks and/or your commute if you

are not driving

- Taking regular stretching breaks
- Breathing breaks

I hope that this chapter has given you a sense of the types of things you can do to support yourself while at work and after work! If you need an advocate to help you negotiate support at work, then please contact a local Citizens Advice Bureau or disability agency. Do not be afraid to ask for help.

Managing Emotions with Chronic Illness

In my travels through the research around Fibromyalgia and CFS, I keep coming across references to depression. Some doctors will try to say that Fibromyalgia is really depression.

I do have to confess that I work hard to stay away from the "black dog." It is hard to stay positive in the face of continual pain and soul crushing fatigue.

There's no way to describe what it's like living with this. There's no way to describe that I feel like I'm continually letting down my husband and children or that I feel trapped by what I need to do to minimize my symptoms.

I get sad and I feel angry.

The only person who suffers when I do too much is me. The increase in pain and fatigue is hard to take when it's already hard.

The balance is difficult.

I used to find it tricky to assess what was reasonable, but I have since learnt that all of my feelings are reasonable and acceptable. As long as I have safe outlets for managing the big emotions and seek help when I really need it.

Also know that, with the kinds of symptoms we are dealing with, it is reasonable to struggle with emotions. Of course, we are sad when we are continually sore or miss out on fun things. Of course, we are happy when we feel well. It is wholly reasonable to grieve. And grieving with a chronic illness is not linear. Just when you think you have a handle on it, something will bring it all up again. And it's okay. If you're focusing relentlessly on how sad you feel or lose the will to fight or just feel generally quite bad, then please seek help. You don't have to face it alone. You don't have to feel miserable.

Journaling has been a go-to tool for me since I was very young. I write through my fears, hopes, dreams and experiences. My journals from when my health was at its worst are full of hope, plans and dreams. There are also parts that are bleak. Being able to work through those emotions is helpful.

Finding the balance between positivity and realism is tricky and one I try to mindfully manage in what I say, write and think.

I also think that finding a suitably experienced and qualified counsellor could be a useful addition to our whole life plan. I have tried a few times to find a counsellor that suited me and haven't found the right fit. Being able to share what we are managing, and feeling is part of human connection. One help here is finding those few people that I can talk to. Being able to talk to someone about what I experience, rather than bottling in up, has helped me a lot.

Support

When I was first diagnosed – and for a great many years after – the only person I spoke to who had even heard the term

Fibromyalgia was my doctor. And she not only didn't help me at all, but she also discouraged me from reducing my work hours as she believed I'd be disappointed that I'd still be sore and tired. Boy, was she wrong.

It's only recently that I've had a tiny team and most of them are virtual connections. If there is no one in real life, get a virtual crew. I like the solutions-focused groups because they provide a real sense of not doing it alone. And all of them are fighting as hard as I am and have much to offer in advice. As part of my exclusive members' team, we have an exclusive group where we can ask questions and I share extra information and support. I find this as valuable as the members do! During a challenge I ran a couple of years ago, we started a Facebook Messenger group that continues to this day. We bounce ideas off each other, I share yoga tips, and we generally check in on each other. I am not sure what I'd do without these ladies.

I have had a profound longing to be witnessed, to not be alone. As I found when I had my babies, there was nothing worse than being completely alone, in pain, and exhausted with a screaming baby. Even if the person can't help any of the issues, their presence, especially if it's my husband, soothes me.

My sister and younger brother, Luke, have both lent me a compassionate ear many times. For that I am grateful. Luke has helped me a lot in many different ways. But the thing I am most grateful for is that he always understands my context. It doesn't hurt that he recognises how hard it is to achieve what I achieve each day and regularly tells me. He has also never made me feel like I am not enough or made me feel like I have to explain myself. That is a blessing.

Nothing fills the gap like someone who gets it. I highly recommend connecting with others who are fighting this journey. At the same time, I don't recommend people who are not actively fighting Fibromyalgia and are maybe a little pessimistic. – I would struggle letting someone vent and not being able to suggest anything to help. And listening to the same complaints over and over again would be frustrating. Find what works for you and connect. Especially if you are stuck at home a lot, humans are social creatures. We need each other.

Just know you are not alone. There are millions of us fighting together. Connect. Find fellow chronic illness fighters on Facebook, or in a local meet up.

The Label Problem: Balance and Self-Perception with Chronic Pain and Fatigue

It's the age-old question of functionality vs symptoms. Are we willing to suffer the symptoms in order to do something? For years, I have waited for someone to truly understand what it is I deal with on a daily basis. I have also spent more years than not ignoring it and carrying on because I had no label and no idea it was reasonable – or preferable – to go a little easier on myself.

For the last three years, I have acknowledged my illness and my limitations and worked to both learn about them and conquer them.

But there is a tricky balance here. You don't want to dwell on your pain and fatigue or whatever symptoms you deal with, you don't want to stop doing things you want to do, and you don't want to be seen as the sick person. You do, however, want to know your boundaries.

I acknowledge and respect my boundaries as best as I can, because I have found that I can often overexert myself and I then pay for it. As my only advocate, I have to pay attention. It can be hard for other people to grasp what it is to struggle through a day or, worse, to be stuck in bed in extreme pain, fatigue, and panic.

Everything I do, I do to stay away from being unwell. I guess, because I look healthy and because I achieve so much, it is hard for someone, even someone who witnesses my everyday life, to grasp the fact that I could be one bad call away from a flare up. So when I compromise and stay out late, I am compromising my energy and my experience of wellness. Even if I am not in bed the next day, my pain could be worse, my fatigue will probably be increased, and that day becomes a day that I am not living but merely coping t.

On the flip side of that, I do tend to protect myself a little too much. I appreciate it when my husband can remind me to do something I think may be a little too out on the cost/benefit scale because I can get it wrong. I can overestimate the cost and underestimate the benefit. But there needs to be recognition that I can't stockpile energy and it takes more than one night to make up for depleted energy levels.

So, it comes back to a tricky balance. You need to acknowledge your illness/boundaries, but you also need to try to learn where you can push back. This can be difficult with an unpredictable illness like Fibromyalgia and Chronic Fatigue, but when you're pushing back includes achieving something you're passionate about, it is so worth it. Then, maybe you're not the "sick" person, but the "wise" person.

Parenthood
With Chronic Illness

This is no small feat to have birthed and cared for four small children. It wasn't easy. But I don't regret it one bit. They are so part of my life that all my coping mechanisms must fit around them. But for this section, I'll focus specifically on parenting with a chronic illness. Generally, I am referring to my experience as a mama. But I hope this helps all parents, ones who have a baby physically or not.

Pregnancy

I am so passionate about sharing information about pregnancy and Fibromyalgia that I wrote a book about it. It was an eye-opening experience to write about pregnancy with these illnesses. When I had Noah, there was so little information; it just wasn't a nice experience. When I had Wyatt, there was a little more literature, and I had all my knowledge, hard gained from my first experience. By the time I had Nathaniel, in 2018, I not only had my experience and research, but I had a fantastic group of women in my Facebook group Pregnancy and Fibromyalgia to share the journey with. Please come and join us if you are pregnant or intending to be!

Here are some of my key tips for being pregnant with chronic illness:

- Arm yourself with knowledge
- Get your body into the best place possible before conceiving
- Prioritise rest and sleep
- Nourish your body with good food and appropriate supplements
- Plan for the final trimester, delivery, and the first six month that involves a good support system
- Get a pain management plan in place, discuss with your doctors what medicines you cannot come off, what you can stop taking during your pregnancy, and get your natural pain management mechanisms in place

My experience will not dictate how you experience pregnancy. Some experience a holiday from their symptoms, but I found it far more difficult. It is useful to hear other people's experiences, so you don't feel like you're flying blind. The above-mentioned six tips are the key things you need to know.

I had two crazy labour stories and then two more normal ones. The first was posterior; he was backwards which caused severe back pain for the entire 20 hours. The second had the cord tied around his neck three times which is very unusual. It was 52 hours of misery, but it was misery with an end date and the best pay off. My third gave me two days of pre labour and then just a few hours of active labour with only 24 minutes of pushing. It was intense! My fourth followed the normal pattern of giving birth. I experienced a day of gently escalating contractions that I could continue my day in between, and active labour was over very quickly. It was intense for about three hours. There was around 45 minutes between arriving at the hospital and delivering him.

The one thing that seems to be more common is a flare up after birth. The sleep deprivation, the pain, the 24/7 job that is looking after a baby are all rough, so choose your best support person and use them.

You can read about my nursing post on my blog or in my book, but here's what I will reiterate:

You count.

You are absolutely part of this equation. If nursing hurts too much, if you hate it, if it's not working – you have the right to say no. Your baby needs you more than your breasts. (Yes, breast milk is nutritious and excellent, but not at the expense of the parent.)

It's not all or nothing. You can feed direct, express, top up with formula or do all three. I lasted much longer with my second baby because I utilised all three of these options and it was a much better early parenting experience. With my third I was thankful to exclusively breastfeed past the three-month mark.

One day, one week, one month, one year – it's all success. Go you!

I will believe in each one of these points for the rest of my life. I will never allow a person to contradict these without a firm response. Support people supporting new parents! Please have their back.

Fourth Trimester

After the work of pregnancy, labour, and the first few days, the most beautiful thing you can do for your baby and your body is to rest.

In places like India and Asia, women have a "lie in." For a month, they stay in bed and focus only on the baby and their recovering health.

You can look at this as a fourth trimester to ease you and baby into life.

First and foremost, we need to be more caring towards ourselves. Pregnancy is a difficult time for even the healthiest women. Labour is hard. Adjusting to a tiny needy baby is a real test of endurance. Taking that time and not considering it business as usual is really important, particularly when you have a chronic illness for which pain and fatigue are already an issue. You're likely to flare up post birth. Sleep deprivation is no friend to pain or fatigue.

To give us a fair chance at succeeding in the endurance race that is the first year of having a new baby, let's consider the first few weeks as necessary resting/adjusting/healing time.

Some Useful Tips for the Post-Birth Period

- Consider day and night as feasible sleeping times. Try to arrange it so that you're not reliant on medicines that stop you getting to sleep without them. You may like to distinguish between night and day for the baby, such as daytime feedings in the light, talking and singing, and night-time feedings in dimmer light and quieter.
- Eat as best you can, despite potentially being too tired and sore to feel hungry. Consider smoothies with fruit and vegetables.
- Stay hydrated.
- Resume your pelvic floor exercises as soon as possible. This will help you regain your strength later.
- Let your dad/partner/parent/friend take the baby so you can rest and shower and eat and rest.
- Consider meditation for a nice booster. 20 minutes of Yoga Nidra is worth a few hours of sleep! You can save varying lengths to your phone. Prayer is also meditative.
- If you're breastfeeding, be wary of posture, hydration, and fuel because it takes more energy than you may have.
- If you feel breastfeeding is a kick in the pants after your previous ordeals, as I did with Noah because it was far too painful and exhausting, don't feel guilty. You need to look after this baby and you for a long time yet. Try to sense how much you can cope with before the meltdown. Know that whatever you can give is beneficial. There are multiple options available to you.

- Switch between a comfortable chair/couch and your bed so your body doesn't get too sore from the same position. My best tip for surviving the postpartum period is to learn how to create a safe space, nurse in a side-lying position and sleep or meditate at the same time.
- Jot down notes for memory. I took many photos, videos, and notes that I love looking back at.
- Store up some movies or TV series you might like to watch on lazy days or when you're feeding.
- Have any supplements/medicines that you couldn't have while pregnant and that are safe to take when breastfeeding on hand, so that they're ready for you.
- Don't be too impatient to wean yourself off painkillers too fast. I forced myself off too soon with Noah thinking it was better to be less reliant on medicine, but I was only denying myself perfectly acceptable coping mechanisms.

Tricky Parenting Secret

Do you want to know a tricky parenting secret? It took a while to dawn on me. It doesn't take as much as you think to make a nice day for your kids.

Take a day in 2017 as an example. I was exhausted and my pain levels had been creeping up thanks to the baby waking up six times a night. We went to church. With a baby and a three-year-old; it's not so peaceful anymore and we got frustrated with Noah not being quiet. We know he can't sit quietly for just over an hour, but not yelling would be great.

Back at home, he was frustrating us. We were feeling cabin fever but also the weight of the incomplete housework. The baby wasn't playing ball with napping. I was so tired I felt sick.

But we decided to go out. I wanted to be tired and sore out, instead of tired and sore at home. So, we bundled into the car, drove half an hour, of which the baby slept 25 minutes, and visited a nice beach with a park. Parking was difficult, but we got a 30-minute park, unbundled, and faced the cold but beautiful scene. Noah happily rode his scooter up and down the beach. On the way home, we stopped for chocolate sundaes at a special chocolate cafe.

Noah was difficult to keep occupied as we waited for our order. He was loud on the drive home.

But at the end of the day, as I remembered how frustrating it was to wrangle Noah and the overtired baby and my own issues. While admitting I had a nice time. Noah remembered a great day. He had fun. He remembered the scooter, the birds, the swing, and the chocolate sundaes. And our photos look so great.

My parenting secret is simple: All it took was a park and a treat. And I managed to give that to him, despite pain levels of 5/10 and fatigue levels up at an all-time high.

It was a timely reminder as I worried about my lack of energy and time. I worried that I didn't have enough to split between two kids.

But I do. I continually find reserves I didn't know I had, for their sakes. And my little efforts to keep Noah occupied pay off.

On days where we are housebound by baby and pain levels, Noah is just as happy to bake and colour and ride his digger and snuggle while watching a movie.

So now my definition of a successful day is when I ask Noah, "Did you have a nice day?" And he responds with an emphatic "Yes!"

Parenting Resources

My book *Pregnancy and Fibromyalgia*

Pregnancy and Fibromyalgia Facebook group (I run this)

Fibro Parenting Facebook Group

Being Fibro Mom website

How to Choose
A Treatment Option

Given the fact that there is no one answer for those of us with Fibromyalgia, no magic pill and no set treatment plan, we must find our own way. This is what this whole book is about finding my own way.

So how should you assess treatment options?

- Research
- Check medicines and supplements on Drugs.com website. Look for anecdotal evidence in the form of people with your symptoms or condition who also utilise that option. Patients Like Me and Syndio is a good website for tracking your health and treatments and accessing other's assessments of treatments. Ask someone knowledgeable that you trust. Hopefully, you have at least one doctor in your corner for this. Check for any interactions and side effects. Check its safety in pregnancy if there's a chance you'll become pregnant in the near future.

Cost vs Benefit Assessment

Ask yourself if the intended outcome is worth the monetary investment? Is the intended outcome worth the potential side effects? What are the chances of the potential side effects affecting me?

What's the chance of success? What's the chance of failure? How much might it impact your life? What would happen as a result of it working?

Would you always wonder about it?

Plan for coping with potential side effects. Plan for administering the treatment option.

Document your experiment! This is crucial to assessing the impact. For example, the effects of low dose Naltrexone took more than six months to manifest for me. It was subtle at firs. I might have missed it if I weren't documenting my symptoms. Sometimes you have to stop a treatment to know for sure it was working and be sure to document this too.

Whole Of Life Change: How It Looks Now

I am still in the phase of learning to balance my health with my dreams. The urge to binge on all the things I have missed out on remains. I read around 100 books per year because of all those years I couldn't read for pleasure at all.

My whole life plan is a carefully constructed system that keeps me as well as possible and fully participating in life.

The mission continues, with the creation of this book, several journals to help guide others through symptom tracking and planning with chronic illness, and all of my blog resources. But I am now more focused on moving toward wellness, rather than away from illness.

My dreams lie in enjoying these amazing boys my husband and I made, in revelling in the fact that I get to be married to this man, and hopefully, in helping others learn to live well despite their circumstances.

I hope I make a difference in the lives of those that intersect with mine. I hope I always know what's important. I hope I always fight for my right to be well. I hope my story helps you.

Resources:
Facebook Groups, Books, Websites, Articles

- Drugs.com website
- Deep-heat.co.uk website
- What Works For Fibromyalgia Facebook Group
- LDN Got Endorphins (Low Dose Naltrexone) Facebook Group
- Fibromyalgia and Muscle Pain: Your Guide to Self-Treatment (2015) by Leon Chaitow ND, DO (book)
- From Fatigued to Fantastic! (2021) Jacob Teitelbaum, MD (book)
- The FibroManual: A Complete Treatment Guide for You and Your Doctor (2016) by Ginevra Liptan, MD (book)
- Suffered Long Enough: A Physician's Journey of Overcoming Fibromyalgia, Chronic Fatigue and Lyme (2014) by William Rawls, MD (book)
- The Fibro Fix: Get to the Root of Your Fibromyalgia and Start Reversing Your Chronic Pain and Fatigue in 21 Days by Dr David Brady
- Fed up With Fatigue website
- Being Fibro Mom website

- ProHealth website
- LDN Research Trust website
- History of Fibromyalgia (2013) by Dr Ananya Mandal, MD (article)
- What is Fibro Fog? - Fibromyalgia and Cognitive Dysfunction (2013) by Dr Ananya Mandal, MD (article)
- 11 Ways to Beat Fibro Fog (2012) by Beth W. Orenstein (article)
- Syndio Health (website) (www.syndiohealth.com)

Acknowledgements

Thank you:

Luke, for your tireless hours of editing, formatting, and designing. This book would not have been completed were it not for you. And more importantly, thank you for being excited with me about my dreams and creations.

My husband and my children, Noah, Wyatt, Nathaniel, and Everett – the lights of my life, the loves of my life, the reasons I fight. I'm not one for sentimentality but I love you more than I can express. This, and everything I do, is for you. Thank you.

God. My faith was the only thing that kept me putting one foot in front of the other as a young woman suffering severe pain and fatigue with no one to understand. Without that, I doubt I'd be here now.

About the Author

Melissa Reynolds is a mama of four beautiful boys. She is also a content creator, accessible yoga teacher, and chronic illness advocate.

For nearly a decade she has shared her journey to better wellness despite chronic pain, fatigue, and insomnia on her blog (www.melissavsfibromyalgia.com). In addition to over 300 blog posts and 200 YouTube videos, she has written three books, four journals, a workbook, and several courses.

Melissa lives in Auckland, New Zealand, with her husband, four children, and her dog, Harry.

Before You Go

I hope this book has helped you. If you want to connect with me, scan the codes below:

My blog

This page has extra goodies for you that were mentioned in this book.

My YouTube

My Instagram

@melissareynolds

And could I ask you a favour? Could you please put a review of my book on Amazon and Goodreads? Your review will help others who need information about fighting Fibromyalgia find it.

Melissa's Other Books

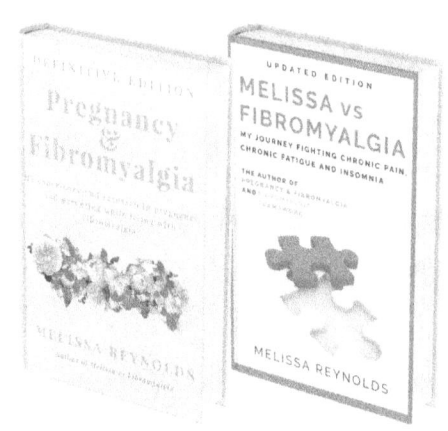

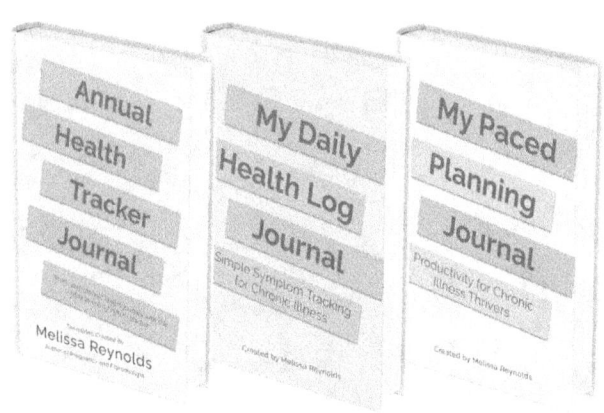

References

Potential Causes

Jane Middleton-Moz & Lorie Dwinell. (2010). *After the Tears: Helping Adult Children of Alcoholics Heal Their Childhood Trauma.* Simon & Schuster.

V. J. Felitti, R. F. Anda, D. Nordenberg, D. F. Williamson, A.M. Spitz, V. Edwards, M.P. Koss and J.S. Marks. (1998). *Relationship of Childhood Abuse and Household Dysfunction to Many of the Leading Causes of Death in Adults.* The Adverse Childhood Experiences (ACE). Retrieved from: https://pubmed.ncbi.nlm.nih.gov/9635069/

What Are These Syndromes?

J. Ahlhamer, J. Lucas, C. Zelaya et al. (2016*). Prevalence of Chronic Pain and High-Impact Chronic Pain Among Adults* — United States, 2016. MMWR Morb Mortal Wkly Rep 2018;67:1001–1006. DOI: http://dx.doi.org/10.15585/mmwr.mm6736a2

Mayo Clinic Staff. (2021). *Fibromyalgia.* Retrieved from: www.mayoclinic.org/diseases-conditions/fibromyalgia/symptoms-causes/syc-20354780

Ernest Choy et al. 2010. *A patient survey of the impact of fibromyalgia and the journey to diagnosis.* Retrieved from https://www.ncbi.nlm.nih.gov/pmc/articles/PMC2874550/

Fitzcharles & Boulos. (2003). *Inaccuracy in the diagnosis of fibromyalgia syndrome.* Retrieved from https://pubmed.ncbi.nlm.nih.gov/12595620/

Inanici and Yunus. (2004). *History of Fibromyalgia.* PubMed. Retrieved from https://pubmed.ncbi.nlm.nih.gov/15361321/

National Fibromyalgia & Chronic Pain Association. (n.d.). Prevalence. NFMCPA.
Retrieved from https://www.fmcpaware.org/fibromyalgia/prevalence.html

J.G. Travell & D.G. Simons. (1988). *Myofascial Pain and Dysfunction. The Trigger Point Manual: Upper Half of Body, 2nd edition.* Lippincott, Williams & Wilkins, Baltimore.

Mayo Clinic. (n.d.). *Myofascial Pain Syndrome.* Retrieved from mayoclinic.org.

I. Kushner, M.D., Z. Issac M.D. (section editor), & M. R. Curtis M.D., M.P.H. (deputy editor). (2018). *Overview of soft tissue rheumatic disorders.*

M. J. McAllister, PsyD. (2013). *What is Central Sensitization?* Retrieved from https://www.instituteforchronicpain.org/understanding-chronic-pain/what-is-chronic-pain/central-sensitization

What Can I Do? Building Your Toolkit

Arthritis Care Res. (1995). *Self-efficacy, pain, and physical activity among fibromyalgia subjects.* doi: 10.1002/art.1790080110.

S. P. Buckelew, S. E. Murray, J. E. Hewett, J. Johnson & B. Huyser. (1995). *Self-efficacy, pain, and physical activity among fibromyalgia subjects.* DOI: 10.1002/art.1790080110. Retrieved from https://pubmed.ncbi.nlm.nih.gov/7794981/#:~:text=Results%3A%20Higher%20self%2Defficacy%20was,pain%20and%20physical%20activities%20impairment.

Pacing and Boundaries

Anne Leppert. (n.d.). *Controlling Symptoms Through Pacing.* Retrieved from http://www.cfsselfhelp.org/library/control_through_pacing

ME/CFS & Fibromyalgia Rating Scale. (n.d.). Retrieved from http://cfsselfhelp.org/cfs-fibromyalgia-rating-scale

The Foundation Upon Which All Is Built: Sleep

Dr Ginevra Lipton, MD. (2016). *The Fibro Manual.* Random House Publishing Group.

Casey Thaler. (n.d.). *8 Tips for Better, More Effective Sleep.* Retrieved from https://blog.paleohacks.com/how-to-sleep-better/

Central Sensitivity/Overactive Nervous System

Dennis W. Dobritt, DO, DABPM, FIPP. *Fibromyalgia - A Brief Overview (a presentation)*. Retrieved from www.michigan.gov/documents/mdch/fibroacpsm_246421_7.pdf

Dr David Hansom, MD. (2016). *Back in Control*. Vertus Press.

Low Dose Naltrexone:
The Medicine That Has Changed My Life

Ethan B. Russo. 2016. Clinical Endocannabinoid Deficiency Reconsidered: Current Research Supports the Theory in Migraine, Fibromyalgia, Irritable Bowel, and Other Treatment-Resistant Syndromes. 1(1): 154–165. doi: 10.1089/can.2016.0009.

J. Younger, L. Parkitny, & D. McLain. (2014). *The Use of Low-Dose Naltrexone (LDN) as a Novel Anti-Inflammatory Treatment for Chronic Pain*. Retrieved from ncbi.nlm.nih.gov/pmc

UAB, College of Arts and Science. (n.d.). *Current Projects*. Retrieved from https://cas.uab.edu/

Dr. J. Carnahan. (2015). *Low Dose Naltrexone: The Treatment You've Never Heard Of*. Retrieved from https://www.jillcarnahan.com/2015/12/19/low-dose-naltrexone-the-treatment-youve-never-heard-of/

Stephen Dickson, Pharm. (2020). *How Long Does Low Dose Naltrexone Take to Block the Body's Receptors*. Retrieved from https://ldnresearchtrust.org/how-long-does-low-dose-naltrexone-ldn-take-block-body%E2%80%99s-receptors

Meditation: Multiple Birds With One Stone

S. Aliano. (2020). *Meditation: A Pathway to Pain.* Retrieved from https://www.practicalpainmanagement.com/patient/treatments/alternative/meditation-pathway-pain-relief

My Favourite Tool Ever: Yoga Nidra Guided Meditation

Kamini Desai, PHD. (2017). *Yoga Nidra: The Art of Transformational Sleep.*

E.N. Moszeik, T. von Oertzen & K.H. Renner. (2020). *Effectiveness of a short Yoga Nidra meditation on stress, sleep, and well-being in a large and diverse sample.* Curr Psychol Retrieved from https://doi.org/10.1007/s12144-020-01042-2

Yoga for Fibromyalgia: It's Not What You Think

Joe Miller. (n.d.). The Benefits of Yoga on the Parasympathetic Nervous System. The Nest. Retrieved from http://woman.thenest.com.

J. W. Carson, K. M. Carson, K. D. Jones, R. M. Bennett, C. L. Wright & S. D. Mist. (2010). *A pilot randomized controlled trial of the Yoga of Awareness program in the management of fibromyalgia.* Retrieved from https://www.ncbi.nlm.nih.gov/m/pubmed/20946990/

J. W. Carson, K. M. Carson, K. D. Jones, R. M. Bennett, C. L. Wright & S. D. Mist. (2012). *Follow-up of yoga of awareness for fibromyalgia: results at 3 months and replication in the wait-list group.* Retrieved from https://www.ncbi.nlm.nih.gov/m/pubmed/22751025/?

i=2&from=/20946990/related

D. Sharan, M. Manjula, D. Urmi & P. S. Ajeesh. (2014*). Effect of yoga on the Myofascial Pain Syndrome of neck*. Retrieved from https://www.ncbi.nlm.nih.gov/pmc/articles/PMC4097917/

N. Vallath. (2010). *Perspectives on Yoga Inputs in the Management of Chronic Pain*. Retrieved from https://www.ncbi.nlm.nih.gov/pmc/articles/PMC2936076/?report=reader

How I Use Gentle Exercise As A Tool

A. J. Busch et al. (2011). Exercise Therapy for Fibromyalgia. Retrieved from https://pubmed.ncbi.nlm.nih.gov/21725900/

My Physical Therapy of Choice: Physiotherapy and Acupuncture

J. C. Deare et al. (2013). *Acupuncture for Treating Fibromyalgia*. Retrieved from https://pubmed.ncbi.nlm.nih.gov/23728665/

All I Had For A Long Time: Amitriptyline

L. Chaitow, ND, DO. (2015). *Fibromyalgia and Muscle Pain: Your Guide to Self-Treatment*.

The Trick With Supplements

Dr. Axel. (n.d.). *8 Natural Ways to Overcome Fibromyalgia Symptoms*.

K. L. Richards. (2011). *8 Energy-Boosting Supplements for Fighting Fibromyalgia Fatigue.*

Fibro Daze. (2014). 14 Supplements That May Help Fibromyalgia.

Dr. Jacob Teitelbaum. (2013). The Fatigue and Fibromyalgia Solution. Avery.

Amino Acid Supplementation

D. S. Silver & L. Gebler. (2016). Nutritional Management of Fibromyalgia. Retrieved from http://www.archivesofmedicine.com/medicine/nutritional-management-of-fibromyalgia.php?aid=9131

L. Ehler. (2022). *Treatments for Fibromyalgia: Amino Acid Therapy.* Retrieved from https://www.living-smarter-with-fibromyalgia.com/treatment-for-fibromyalgia-amino-acids.html

J. Teitelbaum, G. Morello & S. Goudie. (2020). *Nutritional Intervention in Chronic Fatigue Syndrome and Fibromyalgia (CFS/FMS) A Unique Porcine Serum Polypeptide Nutritional Supplement.* Retrieved from https://openpainjournal.com/VOLUME/13/PAGE/52/FULLTEXT/

Headaches, Migraines, and Fibromyalgia

D. A. Marcus, C. Bernstein & T. E. Rudy. (2005). *Fibromyalgia and Headache: an epidemiological study supporting migraine as part of the*

fibromyalgia syndrome. Retrieved from
https://pubmed.ncbi.nlm.nih.gov/15902517/

Dr. R. Moghim. (n.d.). *Fibromyalgia Chronic Headaches Causes, Symptoms, Treatments*. Retrieved from
https://coloradopaincare.com/blog-fibromyalgia-chronic-headache-causes-symptoms-treatments/#:~:text=In%20more%20than%20half%20of,experience%20intensely%20painful%20migraine%20headaches.

The Brain (Fibro) Fog

Fibro Fog: Sleep, Brain Dysfunction Likely Culprits for Cognitive Difficulties Associated with Fibromyalgia, Arthritis Foundation web.

The Fibromyalgia and Food Conundrum

S. Harvey. (2016). The Whole Health Life.

What I do: Morning Stiffness

Fibromyalgia Symptoms website. Morning Stiffness and Fibromyalgia.

Roger Chu, PhD, Lac, QME. (n.d.). *10 Tips to Relieve Morning Stiffness*. The National Fibromyalgia and Chronic Pain Association website.

Working With Chronic Pain and Fatigue

A. Meister & V. Woolfrey. (2021). *How Managers Can Support*

Employers with Chronic Illnesses. Retrieved from
https://hbr.org/2021/02/how-managers-can-support-employees-with-chronic-illnesses

www.ingramcontent.com/pod-product-compliance
Lightning Source LLC
Chambersburg PA
CBHW060253290526
45789CB00001B/316